MIDNIGHT DEMONS:
MY SUICIDAL CAREER WITH MENTAL ILLNESS AND
CAUDA EQUINA SYNDROME

BY:
G. COLLERONE

Midnight Demon

Copyright © 2014 G. Collerone
All rights reserved.
ISBN: 149430886X
ISBN-13: **978-1494308865**

Midnight Demon

Acknowledgements:

I would like to acknowledge a few people for without their support, this book would not be possible. I thank Dr. David A. Jobes, PhD for his consent and encouragement to write about his work so that more people can benefit. I gratefully acknowledge Konrad Michel for his consent of the Aeschi model. To Michelle Linn-Gust for always being there. She has been the inspiration behind the book and my trusted friend. Without her support, this would just be a few pages of words with no meaning. To my dear friends Duane Smith, Tom Tulk, Guy Davies, Karen Williams, Sue Saumure, and the members of the Cauda Equina Syndrome Support Group, who have encouraged me to write this book and been there every step of the way during my recovery. To my psychiatric treatment team, whose support I needed most to wrestle with the demons that almost prevented this work from happening. Lastly, I thank Dr. Edwin Shneidman for without his work, suicidology would not exist. He is no longer with us, but I know he is "with" us.
Special thanks and acknowledgement to my editor, Kim Young.

Midnight Demon

Table of Contents

1. Introduction
2. My Suicidal Career
3. First Serious Suicide Attempt
4. Beginning Of Cauda Equina Syndrome
5. Life With Cauda Equina Syndrome (CES)
6. The Road With New Therapist
7. CES Returns
8. You Learn To Live With It
9. Things Get Out Of Hand
10. Intro To Psychiatrist
11. Where I Am Meant To Be
12. Blog Post: About Aeschi
13. Aeschi
14. Mentioning Of Suicide, Therapist Panics
15. Gender Identity
16. Mourning Loss Of Self
17. Blog Post: Facades 09-23-2013
18. Why I Find Myself Suicidal
19. Blog Post: What Do You Say?
20. Voices And Other Musings
21. Grief
22. My Therapist
23. Start Of Suicidal Career: The Beginnings
    23a. Daily Living Activities
24. Hodgepodge Of Blogs
25. Whenever I Have This Pain, I Freak Out
26. Battles With Self
27. About Hospitals
28. Old Research Journals: Blog Post
29. The Consultant
30. Suicide: My Security Blanket

Midnight Demon

Introduction

This book is a culmination of two illnesses, in one person, that exasperate one another. The first illness is a mental illness, and the second is Cauda Equina Syndrome. The end result is that the person dealing with both of these is constantly thinking of killing himself. I have tried to deal with both illnesses in a dignified manner, but you cannot do that with Cauda Equina Syndrome. When it strikes, it hits you hard and you are left feeling powerless about anything you were able to do before it struck. Ordinary tasks such as cooking and cleaning are arduous after getting Cauda Equina Syndrome. So is the simple task of bathing/showering. And whatever you were able to do before is no longer. If you were working when this happened, your job might be compromised or, worse, you can never go back to it. It depends on the severity. You might try to rejoin the workforce, but it only brings you pain and misery. Throw in a lifetime of severe depression and psychosis and you have a whirlwind of suicidality.

I wrote this book, albeit haphazardly. I didn't have a beginning, a middle, or an end in mind. It started off as a couple of my blogs put together, then some writing that morphed into chapters. Next thing I knew, there was enough substance to form a book. It was hard work and, at times, I had to take a break from it because the memories it stirred up were powerful enough to try and send me over the edge. Writing about my suicide attempts were the hardest and most personal. Although this book deals mostly with my suicidality, it also deals with my chronic pain that has sometimes lead me to be suicidal.

Like I said before, there are a couple of illness that I deal with...mental illness (depression that lead to hypomania or psychosis, sometimes both) and Cauda Equina Syndrome. We all have experienced depression at one point or another. I suffer from it constantly. It is unremitting and has brought me to be suicidal more times than I can count, more hospitalizations than I can count, and more suicide attempts than I can count. This book is all about being a suicide attempt survivor for if I didn't survive my attempts, there would be no book. I have included a couple of blogs that I have posted on my website.

This book is called Midnight Demons because, for me, the night-time hour is when the demons come out. It is when the pain, physically and psychologically, is worse. Mix them together and I have written more at night than I do during the day. During the day, it is hard to gauge the level of pain you feel so you go about your business doing your normal routine, whatever that may be. But in doing so, you are causing the pain demons to build up. You put on the façade of being okay and not being depressed. Or you don't and just have a grumpy day. But no matter what you do, the demons come out at the end of the day. And the demons are my suicidality. It is the one responsible for my suicidal thoughts and feelings because my psychological pain is unbearable.

Cauda Equina Syndrome is a neurological medical emergency that happens when the cauda equina (horse's tail) nerves, which are located in the lower back and start when the spinal cord ends (typically T12/L1), become compressed. This can happen one of two ways. First, through trauma, such as a fall or car accident, that resulted in a ruptured, herniated disc, or broken fragments of the vertebrae to go into the spinal canal. Second, by a tumor. The window of recovery from this condition is between 24-48 hours. If surgery is not done within that time frame, nerve damage could become permanent. It takes a long time for these nerves to heal and, even after twelve years being post-operative, I am still recovering. I like to refer to this condition as post-Cauda Equina Syndrome because most doctors don't know what to do after the surgery has been done to treat the pain you are still in. They think that once the surgery is over, you should be fine and be able to get on with your life. I am here to tell you that is not the case, at least not in the beginning. I was unfortunate enough to get this condition twice so my progress was hindered, which ultimately lead to my disability.

Midnight Demon

There are varying levels of CES. Some have the textbook case of it, which involves everything from the waist down. Loss of control of bowels and bladder, numbness in the lower legs (either one leg or both), foot drop, loss of sexual sensation, loss of saddle area feeling, and numbness of the lower back are all common. But, not all cases have all these symptoms. Some may have the foot drop and lower extremity problem. Some may have the extremity and bowel/bladder problem. Either way, after surgery you can be better or worse, depending on the skill of the surgeon and the time it took to get the surgery. I was fortunate to have a quick diagnosis and surgery right away, but I am still left with nerve damage in my foot and ankle. My bowels and bladder don't work right, especially after my second diagnosis. I cannot feel myself when I have a bowel movement if the stools are soft. I sometimes have urine retention with overflow of the bladder. "Overflow" is just a fancy word for leaking. I don't know that I am full most of the time and it takes a long time for the signal to reach my brain to tell me that I have to go.

I also talk about what has helped me with dealing with my suicidality, such as the works of a few psychologists that are well-known suicidologists. I write about their work to spread the word and to give it some meaning because without it, I am afraid that more people will die by suicide. Their work is cited in the back of the book.

I must stress that I am not a medical or psychological professional. The accounts, opinions, and descriptions in this book (unless specified elsewhere) are my own. If you believe you have depression, Cauda Equina Syndrome, or are contemplating suicide, please seek professional help immediately.

Midnight Demon

My Suicidal Career

I write about this not in the sense that Ronald Maris created it, as that would be a completed suicide and I am far from being dead. But my relationship with suicide is a long one, from the time I was eight up until now. It is a struggle I deal with on a constant basis. It, along with my depression, makes life very unlivable for me. I plan my death in so many ways, yet I am unable to act on it.

When I was younger, I had no problem acting on my impulses to kill myself. But then protective factors, such as my niece and nephew, entered my life and I couldn't bring myself to go ahead and do it. The loss would be too great for them. I couldn't imagine what my sister would say to these young kids who adored me. They were my saving grace whenever I had a bad day and really wanted to end my life.

Then, chronic physical pain entered my life and made the balance of protective factors seem out of reach. Protective factors are things that help guard against suicide. It is the reason for living. For example, having kids or a spouse can be a protective factor in preventing suicide because you don't want to hurt that person. I felt that I had to ignore these factors in order to let myself get into the suicidal frame of mind. And I got there several times in the last few years. During one of these episodes, I had a friend call me every single day for a week until the storm had passed. I had therapy several times a week. Nothing stopped the physical and psychological pain that I was feeling. And when the pain got worse, so did the suicidal feelings. The feelings turned into plans that never were executed. This is the story of how it evolved and how a few suicide attempts lead to more hospitalizations than I can count.

I first thought about killing myself at the age of eight. I don't remember the particulars, but I thought it would be a grand idea not to be alive anymore. It got worse when I was nine. I really thought that ending my life was the answer to my problems. I hated myself because I felt like I was a burden to my family. I felt I had let them down somehow. I started planning my death at my birthday that year because I couldn't stand the pain of living anymore. But, for some reason, the age of ten had a significance for my family and my mother was throwing a big party. I don't know why she was throwing the party and making a big deal out of it, but I figured I might as well stick around and see what I got. I was disappointed that I didn't get a tape recorder that I wanted. I didn't try to kill myself that day, but I did try later that year when I had an argument with my mother. To this day, I don't even remember what we were fighting about. I just told her I wish I was dead and went to my room to try and kill myself. I placed a pillowcase over my head and prayed for death to come take me away. It didn't work. The pillowcase was too porous. I was left crying in my room for what seemed like hours. I don't recall if my mother ever checked on me. I hated my life from then on. Suicide was always on the back burner for me.

This is a book detailing my career in suicide and the journey I took to deal with it. There have been a couple of close calls, but nothing recent, although I still feel the need to kill myself at times. But I do not act on my thoughts. I have attempted suicide many times and, according to all the statistics, I should be dead. The one study that I am often in awe of is the one where they found that suicide attempt reactions often predicted future suicide deaths. I am in that category of not wanting to live, yet I am still here. I am the outlier. And I hate being the outlier.

This story is my life. It centers around my suicidality and the works that helped me get through it. Without finding the American Association of Suicidology, the works of Edwin Shneidman and David Jobes, I doubt I would still be around to talk about my life in this way. There are concepts from these people that I hope to explain in layman's terms so people know about them because they have had a deep impact on trying to keep me alive.

The first is Edwin Shneidman's conception of the word "psychache". It is a word used to describe

Midnight Demon

psychological pain, which is defined as the combination of hopelessness, unbearable despair, loneliness, guilt, worthlessness, unbearable anguish, intolerable pain, and helplessness one feels when in deep despair. It is the pain one feels that is deep within you when contemplating your life. His other concept, The Twenty Frustrated Needs, is another brilliant sign of what constitutes suicide. They are:

ABATEMENT: The need to submit passively; to belittle oneself.
ACHIEVEMENT: To accomplish something difficult; to overcome.
AFFILIATION: To adhere to a friend or group; to affiliate.
AGGRESSION: To overcome opposition forcefully; fight, attack.
AUTONOMY: To be independent and free; to shake off restraint.
COUNTERACTION: To make up for loss by retrieving; get even.
DEFENDANCE: To vindicate the self against criticism or blame.
DEFERENCE: To admire and support; praise, emulate a superior.
DOMINANCE: To control, influence, and direct others; dominate.
EXHIBITION: To excite, fascinate, amuse, entertain others.
HARMAVOIDANCE: To avoid pain, injury, illness, and death.
INVIOLACY: To protect the self and one's psychological space.
NURTURANCE: To feed, help console, protect, nurture another.
ORDER: To achieve organization and order among things and ideas.
PLAY: To act for fun; to seek pleasure for its own sake.
REJECTION: To exclude, banish, jilt, or expel another person.
SENTIENCE: To seek sensuous, creature-comfort experiences.

SHAME-AVOIDANCE: To avoid humiliation and embarrassment.
SUCCORANCE: To have one's needs gratified; to be loved.
UNDERSTANDING: To know answers; to know the hows and whys.

When you have frustrated needs, your thoughts of suicide go up. One feels the need to be loved and nurtured and when that doesn't happen, a certain painful loneliness occurs. According to Shneidman, one must rank these needs so the final sum of all is 100. I have never been able to rank them, but I find that these needs are important in everyday life. He got these needs from another psychologist, Henry Murray, in his famous book Explorations In Personality. The theory is that frustrated needs are a causal factor in suicide. Decrease the frustration and reduce the suicide.

Then you have the ten commonalities of suicide (taken from <u>Suicide As Psychache</u>, p34):

I. The common purpose of suicide is to seek a solution.
II. The common goal of suicide is cessation of consciousness.
III. The common stimulus in suicide is intolerable psychological pain.
IV. The common stressor in suicide is frustrated psychological needs.
V. The common emotion in suicide is hopelessness/helplessness.
VI. The common cognitive state in suicide is ambivalence.
VII. The common perceptual state in suicide is constriction.
VIII. The common action in suicide is egression.
IX. The common interpersonal act in suicide is communication of intention.
X. The common consistency in suicide is with lifelong coping patterns.

Within suicide you have a vocabulary of terms. The list is exhaustive, but I have a few favorites:

Midnight Demon

Constriction is the dichotomized thinking, the "this way or no way" thinking that allows suicide to be the "only" thing they can do.

Hopelessness is the feeling of being lost in hope, that nothing is ever going to change, that things will always be the same no matter what.

Psychache is defined as despair, intolerable anguish, hopelessness, guilt, worthlessness, and unbearable psychological pain. It is like a pain in the heart that no one else can feel. Your heart feels heavy and you feel like a burden because of it. Nothing soothes this pain. No medication can touch it. And suicide seems like the only answer.

Lethality is the degree to which someone is at risk for suicide, whether it be a loaded gun or a few bottles of pills or some cuts on the wrist. This is what determines how suicidal a person is and how they are going to act. If the risk is high and eminent, involuntary hospitalization is called for. If the risk is low, then more contact and assessment is needed.

Press is similar to stress. It is as if the building of the press is similar to the pressure of a volcano ready to explode. It can lead to further perturbation and make things worse.

Perturbation is the need to feel or do something to ease the pressure and unbearable anguish and despair they are feeling, to feel better. It can lead to wanting to do something, but the idea is that you need to do something to relieve the pressure of the feelings on your chest.

Fearlessness is the absence of fear. In this regard, it means that people may be fearless when trying to take their life, like a type of Russian roulette.

Competence is the level of competence to carry out the means for their suicidal plan. Examples include a rope for hanging, gun handling and shooting, knowledge of drugs, etc. High competency is a high risk factor.

There are other vocabulary words that I will use in the course of this book, but these are the ones that I will repeat. I also will talk about the Aeschi model and CAMS (Collaborating Assessment and Managing of Suicidality). These two models are similar in their function as they are at the heart of a good alliance between a therapist and a suicidal client.

I am a multi-suicide attempt survivor. The reasons why I have attempted suicide are many. Mostly it was because I couldn't bear the psychache that was at the sole of everything I did. I had the driving need to feel like I belonged, but I never did. I always felt like I was an outcast. I had very few close friends, and still do to this day. I am not an outgoing person and since I lost my job due to chronic illness, I have become more reclusive. But I also have had severe bouts of suicidality that I have come close to acting on. I first thought about ending my life this year but, because my finances got cut, I can no longer end my life. Until I can figure out the location piece, I doubt I can kill myself. And now I thought I would write a book about my struggles. I know that I am not the only one in the world that feels this way. Knowing that you are not alone is the first step in conquering the demons.

Sometimes the demons held different shapes for me. There were times I became dissociative and felt like a different person was taking control, even though I had a somewhat vague awareness of what was going on. I would get into the pit of the abyss and start writing goodbye letters and notes. Some were long and seemed to go on forever, some were short and to the point. I would then fall asleep and didn't realize I sent them until the next morning when people were alarmed. I seriously thought I was writing them to ease their pain, and had no idea I was causing worry. This happened the first time I

Midnight Demon

wrote my psychiatrist an email, thanking her for all her help and that I was sorry that I couldn't go on anymore. I wish I kept a copy of the email to portray what it said, but it is lost forever.

As I went along my suicidal path, there were times I didn't think I was going to make it. In November of 2005, I found myself planning the end of my life and was determined to do so. I could no longer bear it. But my therapist was able to stop me a month before I was going to act on it. I was in college at this time, working toward my bachelor's degree. The following semester, I took a psychometric class. We learned about the different assessments and psychometric tools, such as the inkblot test and the MMPI (Minnesota Multiple Personality Inventory). For our term paper, we had to write about an assessment, or lack thereof, and why. As I was post another suicidal crisis and was still trying to come to terms with my suicidality, I went on the hunt looking for assessments for psychological pain. I had thirty psychological articles on risk assessment and not one of them dealt with psychological pain. I was discouraged until I was able to find one article written by the father of suicidology, Edwin Shneidman. This one paper opened the door to my world of suicidology. I began reading everything this guy had written and found out that there was a professional organization he founded just for this purpose. I had to become a member and did in 2007…first as a student member, then as a full member after I had to quit college. I got the journal *Suicide and Life-Threatening Behavior*, and I was in suicide heaven. It was through this organization that I came across the works of David Jobes.

David Jobes is my idol. I really love his works and he is a great suicidologist. He really gets what it means to be suicidal and, better than that, he wants to help. Most clinicians do not want to deal with suicidality with a ten foot pole. They are afraid of the risks involved, from liability to malpractice to ethical concerns. Dr. Jobes has written about all of this and created a clinical framework to deal with this population. The framework is called CAMS (Collaborating Assessment, and Managing of Suicide). It is a philosophical, yet empirical theory that has helped thousands of suicidal people get out of their thinking and on with their lives. CAMS was developed specifically to modify clinician behaviors in how they initially identify, engage, assess, conceptualize, treat, and manage suicidal outpatients. It is a brilliant concept that is much needed in outpatient therapy because inpatient treatments have gone by the wayside and insurance companies have dictated more on treatment than on clinical matters. The heart of CAMS is the emphasis on a strong therapeutic alliance where counselor and client work closely together to develop a shared understanding of what brings the client to think about suicide. CAMS is similar to the Aeschi model, where the clinician is open to hearing the client's story of why they are suicidal. It is a patient-oriented model rather than a physician-oriented model.

    The CAMS model has an assessment tool called the Suicide Status Form (SSF) and it is used to assess, make a treatment plan, and track suicidal patients. The cool thing about this assessment is that it's multi-faceted and is not restricted to one mode of therapy or type of clinician. It can be used across all disciplines and types of therapists (DBT, CBT, psychodynamic, etc.) As long as there is a willingness to adhere to the principles of putting the client first, that is the first step in the right direction.

    The SSF is a seven page assessment tool that is used to initiate, track, and follow the outcome of suicidality. It was created so people who are suicidal are not lost to follow-up. More is said about this in Jobes's book, <u>Managing Suicide Risk</u>.

    I have used the SSF in my therapy, but I have to confess that my therapist and I never completely followed through with it. We would use the initial and the tracking forms, but never quite got to the outcome phase of the assessment. Because I felt like it was my idea, and she wasn't into changing her style of treatment, it was difficult to follow through. But that is okay because, regardless, I am still here. We mostly use the SSF to assess my psychological pain, reasons for living/dying, and the level of my suicidality, as well as the likelihood of me killing myself.

    I will repeatedly talk about the works of Jobes, Shneidman, and the Aeschi model throughout this book because I think there is not enough awareness of this in the world of psychiatry, psychotherapy, and psychology. And there is even less in the training of therapists and future psychiatrists. It really is a shame that not enough awareness of suicide is mentioned in the course of graduate college training, and it is often left up to the students to figure it all out on their own, if at all. Usually it isn't until a suicide or attempted suicide happens that people have hindsight, and it isn't always 20/20.

Midnight Demon

First Serious Suicide Attempt

The first suicide attempt that I made that was medically serious was when I was eighteen. I had overdosed on medication. Idiotically, I called my therapist, Dr. B, and was sent to the hospital. I was then placed under guard while on the medical unit. I had to be on telemetry because my heart rate was going crazy. After 24 hours, a psychiatrist determined that I needed further care and I was transferred to the psych unit, where I had been before for a few weeks. This was the fourth or fifth admission to this unit in the past two to three months. Prior to that, I had not made any attempt on my life. I threatened I was going to, but I didn't. I just wanted the pain to end. I felt so worthless when I woke up the next morning. My therapist, who was also my psychiatrist on the unit, was plainly pissed at me for not talking to her prior to doing this. I guess she got into some trouble for it. I had never seen her so mad.

I thought this would be no big deal and I would be home in a week or two. Boy, was I wrong. I was there for two months. I couldn't do anything. Anytime I got privileges, I would somehow lose them. Mostly because someone saw me off grounds of the hospital. I wanted so badly to leave the hospital and just die, but they wouldn't let me do that. I was very pissed. I still am. I just didn't want to make it to my next birthday. I wanted to stay at eighteen forever.

My hospital stay started the beginning of November so I spent the holidays on the unit. I was allowed a pass for Thanksgiving, but that turned into a nightmare on my return because I got a stomach virus and one of the bitchy nurses thought I overdosed again. I had to take a blood and urine test to prove my innocence. I hated that nurse with a passion. She was just so mean.

Christmas was spent in the hospital. I was too depressed to go on pass…or if I did go on pass, I don't remember it. I had to be back by a certain time or they would count me as AWOL and would send the cops after me.

I don't remember much about the hospital stay. The staff was nice and helpful. I spent hours talking to my inpatient therapist (not my psychiatrist; we just left out talks for medication issues) and to the nursing staff, but I did not want to get better. I tried to get them to see that I was meant to die, but that just fell on deaf ears. To them, I had some purpose in this world. But I just saw the world as cold and dark and filled with pain. Pain that no medicine could touch.

I gained a lot of weight while I was in there. I was also diagnosed as having PCOS, polycystic ovarian syndrome. It is a syndrome in which cysts on the ovaries interfere with menstrual function. It was a meaningless diagnosis in the psych ward, but they started me on birth control pills because that was the treatment for it. I guess my medication for my psychosis had spiked my prolactin levels and I needed something to control that. I don't know much about the disorder. I just hoped that taking the hormone wouldn't turn me into a woman. That was my biggest fear, but I couldn't tell them that for fear of being committed permanently. I think they knew my transgender tendencies, but they didn't openly acknowledge them.

I spent the holidays in the hospital. It sucked big time. I hated being there and I hated myself for screwing up my plans to kill myself. If I didn't call my therapist for help, I wouldn't have been in this predicament, and I would probably be dead. But as time went on, I went with the system and rules of the hospital. After a while, I didn't feel so suicidal. I still wanted to die, but it was slowly lessening every day. I turned nineteen in the hospital, much to my chagrin. Soon after the holidays, they were talking about discharge and I had no idea what I was going to do. I had no job. I wasn't enrolled in college. I wanted to go to college, but I didn't know where. I still had a scholarship that my high school gave me, unused and sitting in my bank account. Most of the money I got from my graduation was spent. I bought a ton of nothing while in the hospital, mostly snacks and such because, other than groups, what else were you going to do but eat? I had started to eat a little

Midnight Demon

better to lose the weight I gained and started walking the halls of the unit to try to exercise. I just paced back and forth, especially when I was upset. I would pace the halls while listening to my favorite music.

I applied for college while I was in the hospital and got accepted to a two-year. I enrolled in the associate medical assisting program. I got discharged a week before starting. It was the scariest moment of my life. After spending two-and-a-half months in the hospital, I was finally home and on my own. I still had therapy, but I could do stuff like walk outside whenever I wanted rather than when I was told to do so. I could use real utensils and plates. I was still suicidal at times, but I learned to hide it. It was the only way that I was able to leave the hospital. Besides, I still had my therapist who would keep a close eye on me.

Adjusting to life outside the hospital was a little difficult at first. I still had the routine of waking up at seven in the morning, but now I could sleep late without being interrupted. This only lasted for a week as I had college the following week. I figured if I wanted to go to medical college, this was the best way to find out if I truly wanted to be in that field. The first week of class was manageable. I found that most of the classes seemed "easy" for me. The first semester I made the Dean's List. Then I started having trouble, but still maintained a B average. I didn't end up back in the hospital. I was doing well in college and, even though it was sometimes a pain to get to because I had to take a bus, train, and walk several blocks, I enjoyed it. The classes were small and we got to know the professor and other students well. I was still awkward in social situations so I didn't really interact. I just wanted to get the college work done, then go home and study. I rarely stayed to socialize after class ended. This routine increased when I found a part-time job to give me living expenses.

All this time, I was still seeing the same therapist, a psychiatric resident at the hospital. As Dr. B's residency ended, so did our sessions. I then was transferred to a male resident, Dr. S. I liked him. He was like the brother I never had. He was smart, but had no clue about how to connect to people, much less me. Within a few months of therapy, I was again thinking about ending my life and was taking steps toward that goal. I had been a cutter since high school and he just intensified it. I started cutting to deal with the stress of college and the pain of living. I started seeing him after I graduated college and started working in the medical assisting field. I didn't find a permanent job right away. I started working for a temp agency.

In December of '97, I started to deteriorate again. The cutting got to the point where I needed stitches and I became hospitalized for my safety. I managed to get out so as not to lose my job. I was still trying to keep myself together and have an open relationship with this therapist, but it was getting to be more of a hassle each time. When I told him I was planning on overdosing to kill myself and he asked if I was suicidal, I finally said I needed another therapist. That was the breaking point. I had to see another therapist.

He was able to set me up with a therapist at the local hospital where I was working at the time… the medical assisting job hadn't panned out the way I wanted to so a friend found me a job at the hospital as a clinical laboratory assistant.

The new therapist, Donna, was a social worker. She had many years experience and I thought I would finally have a stable therapeutic relationship. I worked with her for ten long months, then fired her after I was upset over an argument with my sister and she wanted to know more about my sister's social history rather than how upset I was. I didn't know what to do at this point. I was working at a stable job and had health insurance for the first time.

For about a month-and-a-half, I didn't have a therapist. It took me a few weeks to finally call the community mental health center and set up an appointment with intake. It then took several more weeks to place me with a therapist. By that time, I think I ended up back in the hospital because I had become unstable and suicidal again.

Midnight Demon

     Marilyn, the therapist at the community mental health center, was also a social worker. At first, she was really hard on me. A new form of therapy called Dialectical Behavioral Therapy (DBT) came out and showed promise for people like me with borderline traits and cutting urges. I thought it was crap and still do. Who wants to list how many negative thoughts they have a day and then count them up? It became more distressing to me to do this than just to know that I had them. Needless to say, this therapist and I disagreed constantly over what kind of treatment I was going to have. She wanted to try something new, I wanted to stick with the old. The therapeutic process was going out the window. It was a very rough year, but I didn't go into the hospital. Because this therapist was there at the center for more than fifteen years, I thought she was the one that I was finally going to have a rapport with, finally having a stable therapeutic relationship. I couldn't be more wrong.

     After almost two years of working together, she told me she was moving on and leaving the center. I was heartbroken. I was so hurt that I didn't want to see another therapist again. I was also angry that it didn't work out this time. I knew it didn't have to do with me, but I couldn't help but feel that I did something to make her want to leave. We were in the middle of some good work and then she leaves! It wasn't fair. But, as much as it hurt, I respected her decision. But I wasn't going to go to the same center after that. It was too hard. I started looking for private therapists thinking that would be better and then I wouldn't be having a new therapist every year. This was my ninth therapist over the course of eight years (I had four before I overdosed). Trying to deal with my suicidality and then have a therapist leave was just too much.

     Having a stable therapeutic relationship is the core essence of therapy. Without this piece of trust between two people, the relationship is crap. It won't hold a candle to water. It's all about the connection. What was so painful about this was that there was a connection and, unfortunately, it got severed before it could grow. It hurt. It really hurt. I struggled a lot in my therapeutic relationships because of this. I had 11 therapists and, by this time, I was done with seeking help. I didn't know if I would commit suicide, but I knew that I would not seek help anymore. Unfortunately, I knew I needed help even if I didn't want to go through the hurt again.

To make matters worse, I was in serious back pain. I had herniated a lumbar disc and it was causing havoc. I have never before been in so much pain. Simple things like sitting and walking were difficult for me. Now I was in pain not only emotionally, but physically. Not a good combination when you have suicidal tendencies, but I somehow persevered. I had found a therapist I thought I could work with, but she didn't take my insurance. I thought, You got to be kidding me! I finally thought I had "the one", but I couldn't see her because of insurance reasons. There was no way I could pay out-of-pocket. So I went back to the health center and saw someone that Marilyn recommended. I saw this person, Julie, for three months. She was not the worst therapist in the world, but we didn't click. There was no connection. I tried to get it to work but I realized that it was getting more difficult to work through the turmoil left behind by Marilyn. It was very difficult working through the pain of losing her and all my other issues that brought me to therapy. I was also losing my mind with the back pain.

Midnight Demon

Beginning of Cauda Equina Syndrome

After I stopped seeing Julie, I didn't have a therapist for a month-and-a-half. My job got new insurance in the beginning of the year so I switched to a higher rate insurance that I knew "the one" would take. In January of 2001, at the age of twenty-five, I finally had the beginning of a stable therapeutic relationship. We wouldn't really start working together until a few months later. By mid-January, my mood had dropped so low that I needed to be in the hospital again. Death, forever on my mind, was rearing its ugly head, and I really wanted to go through with it. I went into the hospital to get admitted but there weren't beds available so I got transferred to another facility. Unfortunately, I had to leave against medical advice because my back got considerably worse and I needed to see my chiropractor, which I saw the following day. It was the last time I was ever the same. This was on a Friday, the second of February. The reason I take note of this is because CES is a medical emergency. The longer the nerves are compressed, the longer it takes to recover from.

Twelve hours after seeing the chiropractor, my leg gave out on me. By the next day, I had lost feeling in my leg and I could not stand on my own. I spent the weekend in bed, popping ibuprofen and shuffling to the bathroom. I don't know how I did this as my leg became weaker and weaker with each passing hour. I was alone in my basement bedroom. If I fell, I would have been in big trouble as I didn't have a cell phone. All I had was my cordless phone and I was usually the only one at home.

By Monday, I lost feeling in my toes on my left foot, and my foot just hung there. Later, I would learn that this was called "foot drop". I canceled therapy for the next day because I couldn't walk. I didn't feel better after two days. I had an appointment to see my psychiatrist on that Wednesday so I called to cancel that, as well. I spoke to her and told her I couldn't feel or move my toes. She sternly told me to call an ambulance right away and get to the hospital.

At this time, there was an ambulance diversion going on and I wanted to go to the hospital where I worked so I waited for a friend to come home and take me. It took her and a neighbor to help me down the front stairs. By this time, I was starting to lose feeling in my right foot and toes, as well. I went to the emergency room and waited forever to be seen. All this time, I was in a wheelchair and though I was scared, I still thought all I needed was pain medication and physical therapy and I would be fine. I couldn't have been more wrong. The disc that was troubling me had ruptured and I needed emergency surgery. I developed a rare condition called Cauda Equina Syndrome. By the time they figured this out after my MRI scan, I could not stand on my own at all. My legs were like jelly and both of my feet flopped around. I was so overwhelmed that I said I wouldn't sign the surgical consent until I talked with my psychiatrist. One of the neurology residents paged my psychiatrist at four in the morning. She was the one that told me I had Cauda Equina Syndrome. I had no idea what that was, but it sounded bad. I remember the ER attending saying if the discs went the other way, I would need surgery. Well, I guess my disc went the other way and I was stuck needing emergency surgery. My ordinary back pain turned into a rare condition that happens to a handful of people every year in the United States. And wasn't I the lucky one to be one of those people.

"Cauda Equina Syndrome (CES) is a serious neurologic condition in which damage to the cauda equina causes acute loss of function of the lumbar plexus (nerve roots) of the spinal canal below the termination (conus medullaris) of the spinal cord. CES is a lower motor neuron lesion.

Signs include weakness of the muscles of the lower extremities innervated by the compressed lumbar roots (often paraplegia), detrusor weaknesses causing urinary retention and post-void residual incontinence as assessed by bladder scanning the patient after the patient has urinated.

Also, there may be decreased anal tone and consequent fecal incontinence; sexual dysfunction; saddle anesthesia; bilateral (or unilateral) sciatic

Midnight Demon

leg pain and weakness; and absence of ankle reflex. Pain may, however, be wholly absent. The patient may complain only of lack of bladder control and of saddle anesthesia, and may walk into the consulting room unassisted.

Red flag symptoms for acute Cauda Equina Syndrome (requiring urgent hospitalization) include sciatic leg pain and/or severe back pain; altered sensation over saddle area (genitals, urethra, anus, inner thighs); urine retention or incontinence. If you have these symptoms, medical attention is necessary. Immediate treatment may help to preserve function". (Wikipedia accessed 10/19/2013)

The surgeon came and saw me a few hours later, after I demanded one that was board certified. The residents were nowhere to be found. I was crying, and I didn't know what to do. It was early in the morning, and I hadn't slept in almost 36 hours. I knew if I called my family, they would be in a panic. I didn't want to worry them. I just needed to get through the surgery without worry and then I would be okay, right? I called my friend and thanked her for being there for me. You always see the shows where people didn't wake up or had a bad reaction to the anesthesia so I didn't know if I was going to make it out of surgery. I was scared shitless.

They brought me up to my room and the nurses were so nice. However, if I could have walked, I would have gone out the window. I just wanted to be dead rather than go through what lay ahead of me.

Surgery went fine, except they gave me the wrong antibiotic. This one had no effect on me. They might as well have given me sugar water. Two weeks later, after I was starting to make some progress, I developed a staph infection and had to be taken back to the operating room to clear it out. I was even more scared the second time, as the anesthesia doctors were an intern and the other one a fellow. I was never so sick after the second operation as I was with the first. I couldn't get one word out without vomiting. Zofran, an anti-emetic drug, became my new friend for the next few days. Then I developed complications. With the new, more potent, antibiotics they were pumping into me, my kidneys started to fail, then my liver decided to join in the fun by failing. I tried to do the physical therapy, but I lost so much blood between both surgeries, as they were so close together, I was very weak. The surgeon covering for my doctor said that I would need a transfusion if my hematocrit (blood count) got any lower. It took months for me to get my energy back. Eventually, my kidney and liver functions returned back to normal, too.

    All this time I was in the hospital, I was very suicidal because I was just so upset over everything. I couldn't walk on my own. I couldn't go to the bathroom on my own. I had to have two nurses hold me and another wipe me because I couldn't do it on my own. My legs were still weak. I cried every day from the humiliation and loss of dignity, but the nurses were the best and did what they could to handle my difficulties. During all of this, I had minimal contact with my new therapist. During one of our check-ins, I asked if we could have phone sessions because I was in bad shape. I hadn't had therapy in almost four weeks now. We started talking on the phone weekly. I couldn't believe it. It really helped, though there was at least one session where I fell asleep on her. Chalk it up to the pain medications.

    Two weeks after my second surgery, I was tired of waiting for a bed at a rehab hospital and asked if I could go home. I had some strength back in my legs, though just walking down the hall exhausted me. My right leg was almost back to normal, but I still had foot drop in my left. After some discussion with the team of occupational therapists, physical therapists, nursing staff, and my attending, it was decided that I would have home care. I also still needed to be on intravenous antibiotics for the staph infection so a nurse would have to come to my house daily to give me my dose. Even though I was a medical assistant, intravenous lines were something we stayed away from.

    I was finally sent home on a Friday after being given my discharge instructions, as well as told who was coming to see me for my nursing care and physical therapy. I don't remember if I had occupational therapy visit. The good thing was that I just had to go up one small set of stairs to my house. I would be sleeping on the couch for a while until I gained enough strength to go to my bedroom in the basement because there were some steep stairs to go down. I just wasn't ready for that yet. Because I still had stitches in my back, I was not allowed to shower…just a quick sponge bath. I hated it. After two weeks, I really wanted a shower. I would have taken the stitches out myself if I could have reached behind my back, but I let it be until I saw the surgeon again.

    As my mobility was still an issue and the weather was icy and cold, I only left the house for doctor appointments. I was finally able to walk with a walker. The physical therapist wanted me to walk with forearm crutches, but I said "no". I would progress to a cane or continue with the walker. I only saw her for fifteen minutes a day a few times a week. I timed her by the commercials to my soap operas.

Midnight Demon

Life with Cauda Equina Syndrome

If I was depressed before this happened, it was nothing compared to what happened after I was diagnosed. I really thought I would never walk normally again. I still don't, although you can only notice it when I am really fatigued. The doctors couldn't give me any guarantee that I would be back to my old self. I was on my own in my own healing process, and I was scared and frustrated at the same time. I was finally able to get to my room to get on the computer and do a Google search for my condition. I found some people that had Cauda Equina Syndrome so I joined a support group. That was my saving grace. In 2001, it was only a handful of people, maybe 50 or so. Now it is more than a 1,000 from countries all around the world. So much for being a "rare condition". Most of the members of the group are now from the UK, as the people from the US have dropped off. I have found that people use it for support, to vent their frustrations, and then move on with their lives as best they can. Sometimes we won't hear from people for weeks or months, even years. I am one of the "oldest" members as I have been there since the beginning.

Cauda Equina Syndrome is a complicated syndrome that often brings more questions than answers, more despair than hope. Questions like…When will I have my old body back? Will my back/legs/feet ever be normal again? Will my bowels and bladder ever be normal so I won't have to constantly think about the last time I went to the bathroom? These questions are always in the back of the mind of those that suffer from CES.

Do we recover after this? Anything is possible. Some of us do, some are left with permanent injury because treatment did not happen, was delayed, or it was simply too late. Some have seen recovery after a few months or a few years, sometimes longer than that. Some have gotten worse after surgery, as surgery holds its own risk. The never ending questions are… How do I live like this? How do I live with the pain, the never-ending nerve pain that no narcotic can touch? How can I live when

I can't feel myself having a bowel movement or urinate? How can I live with these dysfunctions? I always have to think of where my feet are because if I get distracted or am too tired, I will trip over them.

It has been eleven years since my first injury, almost six since my second. My first diagnosis happened at level L4/L5. My second was at L2/L3, which was higher and more disruptive. It caused me to be where I am today, disabled to a degree that is more permanent than my initial injury. I do not know if all people that suffer CES x 2 will have what I have. I just know that I hurt, that I can't walk more than a few blocks without debilitating pain, that I have to take medication everyday to live my life with some functionality. Otherwise, I will lose my mind and be in a psych ward, never to be a functioning member of society again.

The past year has been hard to deal with. I finally realized that my initial injury never quite healed the way I thought I did so that left me wide open for injury when I was hit the second time. Now, while I am awaiting accommodations from work, I am doing what I do best…writing my life story so it can be used as a voice.

By being a voice, I can tell people who have been suffering with this condition that they are not alone with this. They have support in their pain and despair. We all have been through the learning to walk again, the painful spasms, the nighttime burning and shock pains that keep us awake, the constant worry of being in pain and seeing endless doctors to find little to no relief. My voice can help answer the questions that arrive at each stage when there seems like there is no recovery in sight.

It is a constant reminder that you are not "normal" anymore. You have your good and bad days, but a good day usually consists of making it to the bathroom on time or having some pain relief, even if it is only for a few hours. A good day might be the day where you just collapse in exhaustion and sleep the day away because you were up the night before in horrific nerve pain that just wouldn't quit no matter how many pills you took before bed. I still

Midnight Demon

have not been able to find the exact right time for taking my doses. Though it has been a few weeks since the 2-4 am pain cycle, that doesn't mean that it won't be back. Most of the time, I think that I have not been feeling too much pain because I have been out of work the last month or so. The pain has become less, but if I happen to walk too much or stand too long, I pay for it at night.

People think that you are fine most of the time because you don't have anything physically wrong with you. I find that to be true because other than my foot swelling up, no one would know that my leg is hurting me so bad that I can't walk far or stand for more than twenty minutes. They might see my ankle/foot orthotic, AFO but that is what helps keep my foot aligned. So far I have not been questioned on this by anyone but, then again, this will be the first summer I will be wearing it. I got it in early November because I do not walk correctly due to the weakness in my foot. Instead of walking heel/toe, up/down, my left foot goes heel and swerve to go back to the toes. It's pulled my muscles and tendons so badly that when they flair up, I am in such agony that all I can think about is killing myself. And this pain is 24/7. It drives me nuts because there is nothing I can do for it, nor is anything I am taking helping it. I am on anti-inflammatories, narcotic pain medication, neuropathic pain medication, and I still am in bone crushing pain. All the tests, MRIs, and x-rays said things were normal. But if I am so damn normal, why am I in so much pain??

Then there is the bouncing game where you go from one specialist to another hoping to get a new treatment, a new diagnosis, or just plain answers, but all they can do is give you no answers and refer you to another specialist. My neurologist is good for this. She sent me to a physiatrist, an orthopedic, and a physical therapist, and they all said they have no idea what is wrong with my foot. They have no idea what is causing the pain, be it from my back or from my foot, which turned out to be a mechanical problem.

I have come to the conclusion that despite my many attempts to find the right doctor for my physical pain, there isn't one out there. My last appointment this week was the last new doctor I will see for a while. I am tired of being put through the tests and the endless questions just to be told this may or may not help, but try it anyway. Seeing as I don't have insurance at the moment, I say the hell with it. I cannot fathom going through something for six weeks that might or might not help and then be told, "Well, at least we tried". Nowhere in the literature did I sign up for that.

Not everyone is the same when it comes to pain. I don't even fit the typical symptoms of what my neurologist diagnosed me with (Complex Regional Pain Syndrome) so how am I supposed to have confidence for six weeks? Did I mention this is a "drug free" program? I am supposedly weaned off my pain medication. No, thank you. I can't function as it is without them. I can't take a shower, go down the stairs, or walk unless I take them. Living with this, Cauda Equina Syndrome, post (CESp) is life altering. Throw in mental illness and you got a time bomb of suicidality you don't even want to think about. Most of my midnight demons come from the pain I feel at 2 am. No doctor sees a patient at 2 am unless you are in the emergency room. Of course, my pain level isn't astronomical at 11:40 am when I see a doctor or my psychiatrist. All I can do is shoot off an email at 2 am and tell them I am hurting. Sometimes I get a response, sometimes I don't.

I'm done with seeing new doctors. As long as my PCP provides me with pain relief, that is all I care about right now. I can barely stand when I get up in the morning and no one understands. I don't understand how the medical profession can know so much science and technology, yet know so little about how to treat pain. I'm just getting fed up and tired that no one listens or cares that someone with a depressive condition already is being made to suffer because of the "ills" of opioid therapy. Granted, there are people out there who have addictions, but these people can be weeded out if the physician just takes a little more effort in listening rather than prescribing just to get rid of

Midnight Demon

the patient. I still long for the day when I can page a doctor at 2 am and tell them I'm hurting because I really think they will then understand that I am not just some nut, but a person who is truly in pain and suffering a great deal. However, that day will never come. I will always be the one to suffer and as long as I do, whether it be physical or mental, I will have suicidal thoughts.

I know that, one day, I will take my life. I think, at this point, I am just too tired to even do that. Yes, too tired and exhausted to take my life, to end the pain and suffering caused by the damage of tiny disc fragments that compressed my spinal nerves for five long days. That was all it took to wreck my life forever. I often wonder if I would have finished my degree by now had CES not entered my life for the second time. I believe that this second occurrence is what truly disabled me, physically and mentally. I have more damage than I had before because a tiny fragment was left on my nerves for 4 days after the surgery to help me when I was losing control of my bladder. That problem was solved but, because of this tiny fragment, I was left with paralysis of my left leg, the leg that is now the bane of my existence.

No one knows much about this Cauda Equina Syndrome, yet no one has suffered from it twice and been "okay". I can still walk, but I am tortured by it every day. Every day, my ankle refuses to flex when I wake up. Now it seems I have to take pain medication just to get out of bed and down the stairs to use the bathroom. However if I have to go urgently, it's screw the pain medication and go one step at a time. This is what my life has become.

Not one doctor in the entire city of Boston wants to help me. Mentally, I can't really complain. I have the best psychiatrist I could ever ask for. But medically, I do not have anyone I can truly trust. People just take it for granted that they will be okay after surgery. But no doctor deals with the aftermath of traumatizing surgery and the pain that comes with it. I am sure if I go to my surgeon today, he will either want to do another one or refer me to a "pain doctor" for an injection in my spine. However, those have not been shown to be useful. They might work in 50% of the patients, but not all and some may even be harmed by this practice. I call it a practice of negligence.

Midnight Demon

The Road With New Therapist

Once I got my walking down pat and the infection under control, I started seeing my new therapist, Bozo (not her real name). We started where the last therapist left off, though she still wanted to talk about my condition and the trauma it caused me. I didn't want to talk about the ordeal I just went through, even though it was still affecting my life. I wanted to talk about my other issues that brought me to therapy, the relationship difficulties I was having with a friend, and work. It was too soon to talk about the "trauma" of losing the ability to walk. I would find that I would still talk about this issue because it ultimately lead to my disability and loss of work. My mental health declined, as well, but I think that if I didn't have chronic pain, I could handle the depression.

I was strapped for cash after being out of work for almost two-and-a-half months so I needed to go back. The trouble was that I went back too soon and it caused a lot of pain. My back pain returned and it wasn't until I was on adequate pain medication that I could do my job without difficulty. This went on for a few months until I started having mood swings. Little did I know that it all had to do with my time of the month. I would be really happy and then crash a few weeks later to the point of being really suicidal. This went on for another few months and after each episode, the depression just got worse and worse. I had to go back into the hospital for medication stabilization, but they put me on the detox floor. I had a nut for a psychiatrist and we fought constantly. This psychiatrist thought that one of the antidepressants I was on was an antibiotic. I didn't have trust in her to treat me after that. Then she wanted me off my pain medication and lied to me saying that as long as I was on them, none of my doctors would treat me, including my primary care doctor that was prescribing me my pain medication. I had been with my psychiatrist since I was seventeen, and my primary care doctor for at least four years. I seriously doubted that both of them would turn me down because I was in pain and took something for it.

After I got out of there, I went to my doctors and found out they were still there for me. My primary still continued to prescribe me my pain medication and life was somewhat good. I vowed never to go back to the unit, even if it was the last one on the planet.

All this caused yet another disruption in my therapy with Bozo. We talked about how bad that treatment unit was and how the psychiatrist was awful. She didn't even know the medication she was prescribing. I knew more than she did. It was sad. This was in July, 2002. I was past the year mark with my therapist and was getting nervous because I knew she was getting married soon. My first therapist that I saw when I was a teen, Maureen, had ended therapy soon after getting married because she decided to move out of state. I repeatedly asked Bozo if she was staying or going. I was terrified that I was again going out on a limb only to have it fall short and have to see yet another therapist. But in the weeks that followed her marriage, she was still there.

Around this time, my friend ended our relationship. I became distraught and started drinking to deal with the pain. I was binge drinking alone in my room so nobody knew I was doing it. Obviously, my depression worsened, but I didn't care. I had to get rid of this pain. During our relationship, she had forced herself on me several times, but because of my nerve injury, things were painful. I tried to get her off me, but she always got her way and no matter how many times I said "no", it was never enough. So I drank to those memories, too. I never talked about them until the moment of writing this. Homosexual rape is rarely discussed anywhere, but it does happen. I am sure I am not the only person that this has happened to.

I blamed myself for this mistreatment. On some level, I knew it wasn't my fault. I just couldn't understand why someone who supposedly loved me would want to hurt and disrespect me. She found someone new and I was on my own again. In the fall of 2002, I started college again. This time, I went

Midnight Demon

back to a four year institution to earn my bachelors. All this time, I was still seeing Bozo.

During the time that I have known her, she moved to different locations. She started out in the middle of Mass Avenue, then moved to the end of Mass Avenue, and finally ended up thirty miles away from me in a town called Framingham. That was all well and good, but I didn't have a car at the time. I still don't. While she was relocating, I was having anxiety about her moving. Though she had assured me Framingham was her last and final stop, I was still hesitant. It's been several years now and she hasn't moved again. She also has a little one so I know she isn't going to be moving anytime soon…I hope!

In 2004, Bozo went on maternity leave. She was still at one of her locations in Cambridge and I got close to her office staff. They shared a picture of when the baby was born. When Bozo came back in January, 2005, I later learned the baby's name. She was born one month before the Boston Red Sox won their first World Series in recent history. For a crazy Boston fan like me, this was more than awesome. As Bozo was away for three months, I had an interim therapist, John, who was more of a sports fan than Bozo. For the first month of therapy, I think we mostly talked baseball and how the season was leading up to a championship. Playoffs have always been a source of excitement for Boston Red Sox fans. People were going nuts. Unfortunately, a girl got killed when to a police officer fired a BB gun into a rowdy crowd of people lining the baseball park. It was a tragic accident as the odds of it happening again were slim to none. People were so hyped up that the city tried to maintain curfew and limit crowds, but it was impossible. The excitement was just too great. It was a good thing that game four of the World Series was held in St. Louis, or god knows what kind of havoc might have occurred. However, that did not stop people from lining Fenway Park at 6:30 in the morning to congratulate the team when they showed up to get their gear. Baseball season was over and every Red Sox fan was joyous. Today, as I watch clips of that game, Foulke flipping to Meintkeiwitz, I still have to slow down and realize it was the final out and the Sox have won the game. I remember it took me a full two minutes to join in the jubilations because I just could not believe that they had won. Foulke didn't drop the ball and neither did Doug. Routine play executed. Game over with the Sox winning and me crying tears of joy. Even as I am writing this, I am shedding tears. It made me very happy to see the eighty-six year curse over with.

Bozo came back from Maternity leave, and she was happy to be back. She didn't quite understand the whole baseball thing, but she was happy that I was happy, at least for a little while. I was glad to have her back. As much as I enjoyed talking with John, sports was the only thing with which we clicked. We didn't talk about much else. Maybe a bad college or work day, but that was about it. I was still having trouble getting around and my moods were still awful, but I was not as suicidal as I was. Also around this time, my psychiatrist decided to put me on a new mood stabilizer which helped. For the first time my psychache…the pain that is defined as the melding of unbearable despair, unbearable anguish, hopelessness, helplessness, guilt, shame, loneliness, and depression…wasn't as bad. I was feeling content. I was stable and then, somehow, things fell apart later that year.

I was in group therapy that Bozo had set up prior to her being on leave. We thought it might give me some extra support while she was away. It was the first time being in a psychotherapy group as an outpatient. The only other time I was in a psychotherapy group was when I was an inpatient. At first, the group leader and I got along. I didn't agree with everything that he was talking about, but what did I know about group therapy? As time went on, my mood destabilized and I felt like I should go back to the hospital. It was the one place that I could go to "reset" myself.

I had also stopped my medication, on my own. Why bother taking it when I felt so horrible? What I didn't expect was to feel worse than I already did. Like other medications before it, the mood stabilizer wore out after a few months, and I was crashing again. The depression got so heavy that I

Midnight Demon

could barely think. I felt like I was walking in mud most of the time. I couldn't stop thinking of ways to kill myself. I always had a plan in my head, and I was thinking about how to execute it.

By September of 2005, I was headed for a breakdown no one saw coming. I told the leader of the group that I needed to be in the hospital and he told me that I didn't. To me, that just meant I had to die and something snapped inside me. I vowed that I was going to end my life so I started planning. I stopped paying my credit cards. I started getting my affairs in order. I stopped talking to my therapist, and she had no clue what was going on. By mid-October, I could hardly wait the next few weeks. My mood was becoming darker, baseball season was over and my beloved Sox had a horrible year, the psychache was so intense that I couldn't breathe. But I still carried on like there was nothing wrong with me. To the outside world, I was cheerful. This is the façade I would continually put on to prevent anyone from knowing what was really going on. I had to put on a happy face to hide my pain.

My therapist and I had this game we played to get things going when I didn't know what to talk about, but I sure as hell was not going to tell her my plans so she could stop me. This pain was going to end and no one was going to stop me from doing it this time. The game we played was twenty questions. She could ask me anything and I had to answer truthfully and honestly. This was because I would open up only under direct questions. I'd rather talk about the weather than what was really bothering me. Except, this time, it backfired on me. Twenty minutes into the session, I was bored and decided to play the game to pass the time. At this point, I was seeing my therapist twice a week and although I could cancel, I found it hard to do. Ambivalence would get me to call and reschedule. My therapist asked, "What is really, really, really, really going on?"

I was floored and remembered laughing. I could not believe she asked the one question I was not expecting. It took me a few minutes to collect myself and then the dilemma started. Should I tell her what I was planning to do? I was so damn torn. I wanted to end my life, but I also did not want to hurt this person that I had been seeing for the past four years. I managed to avoid the question and escaped from therapy that day with my plan intact. I waited a day, then called and scheduled an additional session. I told her everything I was planning to do. Her response shocked me. She started crying! I never had a therapist cry in front of me. It brought the realness of the situation to light. I obviously meant something to her and though I don't recommend every therapist cry when their client tells them they are suicidal, they should at least feel something.

    I was in shock. I didn't know what to do. She didn't want me to kill myself. That was clear. Why did I have to tell her? Now my plans were going to be interrupted, something I didn't want to happen. I wanted my pain to end. I wondered how she knew so I asked. She said that a former supervisor had told her that when the client starts shutting down, something is going on. Great advice, but it sucked for me. I really wanted to die, but here I was with a crying therapist who was pleading for me not to kill myself. I felt numb. I didn't know what I was going to do…so I did nothing.

    In the sessions that followed, we worked on how I was supposed to live. I still wanted to die, but that was no longer an option. I gave her my word and I never break that. To say I was ambivalent was an understatement. I have never been so conflicted in my life. Did I really want to die? Or did I want to live? It was a tough decision. I wanted the pain to end and I knew how to end it. Although I never went through with my plan, I still felt the sting. I went through feeling worthless and feeling like nothing. I couldn't stop the hurt. I still wanted to end the pain, but I couldn't hurt this crazy therapist that cared so much about me. I never once thought about how my suicide would affect other people. For me, it was an internal battle that only I was struggling with. It was my fight. How dare this idiot interfere with that. I was crushed. I had feelings for her, too, although I didn't let on that I did. How to solve this dilemma?

Midnight Demon

My mood had deteriorated. I was clearly suicidal and my therapist knew I needed help, but I didn't want it. I didn't want to go into the hospital because I had to keep up with work and the façade that I was okay. We decided that I would go into partial hospitalization so I could still work, but I had to take the time off from college. I had to explain to the professors that I was sick and then make up the work I was missing.

Partial hospitalization was probably the best thing for me at the time because it was centered on one thing…making me better in a short period of time. It had groups that focused on problem solving and dealing with distress. Although most of the groups were DBT (dialectical behavioral therapy) based, the counselors there didn't ram DBT down your throat. In two weeks, I was feeling a little better and less suicidal, but I was still feeling lost and defeated. The reasons for killing myself were not clear. That was the one thing that I never uncovered. Most of the sessions that I had were focused on my safety. Uncovering why I was suicidal was left to my therapist.

I don't really remember what Bozo and I talked about during this time. I think I permanently blocked it out because it was a painful time for me. But I survived this crucial period. What I didn't expect to do was make it to the age of thirty. Bozo thought this was significant given what I was going through so on my birthday, she had a little party for me. Ever since 2005, she made it a point to celebrate my surviving another year. Like I said before, she's crazy. I have never felt such caring by a professional. I guess we have a special relationship and she initiated what I couldn't put into words.

This experience taught me a few things. First, there is no lying to a therapist about wanting to kill yourself. Lying is not built into my programming and she knew that I would be honest with her. What stunned me was her reaction. I tend to view it as a couple of things. Second, I meant more to her than I realized. I never felt that with anyone in my life up until that point. The third was that the bond between us formed and she was determined to see that I live my life and not take it away from HER. Every single time I asked her why she cared, she always said, "Because of who I am". She was determined to keep me alive, and that has been harder and harder over the years. However, she is the reason that I am here today because she believes in me when I don't believe in myself. She also refuses to let me go through a suicidal crisis alone. She now has the policy of her making appointments that I have to keep no matter what. SHE is the only one that can cancel.

***

In the beginning of the new year, I still was feeling very low and the emotional pain ran deep. I could barely keep things together. My heart felt so heavy. I told my psychiatrist all of this and she could see how much I was hurting. She decided to ask a favor of me. She wanted me to go back on my medication. At this time, I was not taking anything. I had stopped all my psychiatric medication because they were not doing anything. So, as a favor to her, I went back on my mood stabilizer. Within a few weeks, I was feeling much better. I couldn't believe the difference a few pills made in my life. I felt like a different person. The depression was still there, but it was considerably less than it was. I vowed at that point never to stop taking my medication again.

Midnight Demon

CES Returns

Later on that year, I hurt my back again. I'm not sure if it was from picking up my one-year-old niece or from a bumpy road in my '87 Camaro. Whatever it was, I herniated a disc higher up in my spinal canal that required immediate surgery. I couldn't believe I got Cauda Equina Syndrome again. After surgery, I lost feeling in my left leg. Another MRI revealed that a fragment was imbedded in my L3 nerve root. Off to the operating room I went. My surgeon was great, much better than my first surgeon. This time, I knew what I was going to go through to get back on my feet. The first time, it took me a long time to get back what I lost, but now I lost what I had regained. At this time, my ankle reflexes had slightly returned, but after this second surgery, I lost them. It's been many years and they still have not returned. I also slightly lost control of my bladder and bowel function. This made me wish I had killed myself the year before. I did not want to go through the rehab and subsequent pain that recovery was going to bring. But I had the support group to get me through this. To know that you are not alone in the devastating nerve pain and humiliating experiences of a leaking bladder and loss of control of the bowel can be a powerful experience. It brings you closer to people. I have friends all over the world with this condition. It doesn't matter that we have not met in person. For the people that lived in my state, we did have a get together probably a year or two after my surgery. That was the first time I ever met people with this condition and it was wonderful. To share in the experiences we go through and know that you are not the only one has been tremendous.

All through this, my therapist was there for me. I was very suicidal at times. After surgery, I was house bound. I had very strict restrictions on what I could and could not do. One of those was limited stair usage. At this time, my therapist was still in Cambridge. She only had a few stairs, but she refused to let me be seen in person. We resumed our phone sessions because there was no way I could get to her office with my restrictions. She made sure that I followed them so there were no setbacks. It was tough. I hated being cooped up in the house, but there was nothing I could do about it because I needed a walker or a cane to move around.

Although I was sick and weak at times, I still managed to take a class at the university. I didn't do too well, but I was able to scrape by with a C+ in Biology 101. Even after I had surgery, I asked the surgeon if I would be out by Monday so I could take a test. No such luck, but the professor was completely understanding and let me make up the test. Because this was a three hour long class, once a week, there was no way I could sit through it because my restrictions were to only sit for an hour at a time. I didn't want to disrupt the class with constantly having to get up. I was to learn the material on my own. I would severely pay the price in pain if I sat more than an hour.

Midnight Demon

You Learn To Live With It

It doesn't happen overnight. It doesn't happen in a week. It takes some time, but you learn to live with it…except on nights like this when the pain keeps you awake. You think of death as your only way out. You think of what more your doctor could do to ease the pain, but it's midnight and he's not on call anyway. Besides, they don't want to hear you cry in pain. They just want you to live with it. And that is the toughest thing to do.

I have been battling pain since seven tonight, and it's been a trigger for me. CES started when my left leg went out on me and I was left with foot drop. I wasn't told to live with it. I was told that I was going to have surgery for a condition I had no knowledge of. I still don't have complete knowledge of Cauda Equina Syndrome because it varies with every person. Sometimes the right side is affected. Sometimes it is the left. In my case, it was the left. I still have nerve damage twelve years later.

I haven't been told to live with the pain…yet. But you have to or you lose your mind or your life. It is a conscious effort every day to not stare at the bottle of pills or some other weapon of destruction and think, why not? You have to take the walls down piece by piece and build it back up again to block the pain out the best you can. But sometimes, like tonight, the walls fail you and you are in tremendous pain. My foot/ankle/leg are hurting all at once and all I want to do is scream. But I can't because it's after midnight and everyone else is asleep. Thoughts of wanting to amputate run high on these nights. It's a good thing there isn't a chainsaw in here.

Meds working to stop the pain is a joke. They may lessen the pain some, but they do nothing to ease it 100%. At my best, the pain is on the level of 3 on a scale of 1-10. At my worst, like now, it can be an 8-12. So I will have to take a third pain pill to quiet it down, or I won't be waking up at 6:45 like I need to so I can take dear old Dad for his tests.

I hate my leg right now. I should be able to live with the pain, and I will. But not tonight. Tonight I am writing and writing until I pass out because people should know that, despite having surgery for CES, you are still left in pain. It is called nerve pain and it sucks. Nothing eases it except narcotic medications or some anti-convulsion drug. Oh, how I wish I could call my doctor now. I want him to see the veins popping out on my foot, how swollen my ankle is, and how I can't get it down with ice or elevation.

But I have to *live* with this? I can't kill myself? It really sucks when you know you are in so much pain, and you can't end your life because of it. I have too many people I'm responsible for. People say they will miss me. I often wonder if that is true.

My psychiatrist told me tonight to take my meds and get some rest. How am I supposed to do that when I got pain this bad? I keep hearing her telling me to go to bed, but I can't sleep. The pain is just too fucking bad.

I didn't do anything to cause this. I didn't stand too long, I didn't walk too far, I didn't go up and down the stairs too much today. Well…maybe I did, now that I think about it. I went downstairs a few times to empty my recycle bins and get rid of some boxes in my room.

I wish I could just disappear, permanently, where there is no more pain, no more agony, no more depression. But I don't want to be happy all the time. That would be too weird for me. Just being content is all that I want. Content means being neither sad nor happy, but not being miserable, either.

I just want the pain to stop permanently. Then maybe I could live my life a little better. My third dose of meds and an Ativan have kicked in. This is how I live with it, without putting a noose around my neck. I just put my hat on backwards and I write until the meds kick in.

It helps to write. It really does.

Midnight Demon

Things Get Out Of Hand

In the fall of 2008, my psychosis got out of hand and I landed in the hospital once again. It got really bad where the medication that used to control it wasn't working. I was hospitalized for a two week period to get my medication adjusted and then, after a month, I would stop taking it and become psychotic again. This had never happened before. Usually, the medication would work and I would be fine after a month.

I had to quit college for the time being. Trying to read without a voice in my head was becoming difficult, and the anti-psychotics messed with my concentration. It became too stressful trying to keep everything together. At times, I also became delusional where I thought a co-worker was going to kill me. I ended up back in the hospital because the voices became commanding and were telling me to kill myself again. Everything started to fall apart and I was fighting to keep sane. I was working two jobs and there were no breaks between them. I hardly took time off anymore because the hospital took those days away from me. Sometimes I worked fifteen days in a row just so I wouldn't feel anything. At times, it seemed like all I did was work. I hardly saw my family anymore. I was on call with my research job all the time because I was responsible for the freezers and making sure they were in working order all the time. The stress of it all was turning me into a psychotic mess and I didn't realize it.

This went on for more than four years. At one point, I was so unorganized that my psychiatrist hospitalized me involuntarily because I wasn't myself. I had emailed her telling her goodbye as I couldn't handle the pain of living anymore. She knew something was wrong as I've never written her such a depressing, agonizing letter. This was this first time that I had police and firemen come to my house. It was terrifying. I just kept telling everyone I was just depressed and my psychiatrist took it wrong but, in reality, I didn't know what was going on. I fell apart.

A year later, I started having lower leg pain. It started with a sprained ankle that never healed and it brought me to where I am today. I'd never experienced pain like this. It was maddening. I couldn't sleep because the pain was so bad, which meant that I was in a bad mood all day. It was such a difficult time. I must have seen over nine different doctors and specialists, and no one had any answers for me…until a physical therapist saw the way that I walked. She figured out that my foot was turning wrong and was pulling on muscles that it wasn't supposed to.

After a year of this, I decided to make one of my jobs full-time and decided to quit my research job. I thought that would be the better choice for me, but things got harder as I didn't realize there was more walking involved. I would sometimes have to leave work in a wheelchair after my shift. I couldn't stand anymore and if I did too much, I sometimes would end up in the emergency room because the pain was so bad. Still, no one knew why my leg was swelling and in pain. X-rays and MRI's revealed nothing structurally wrong with my leg, ankle, or foot. The result from my neurologist was Complex Regional Pain Syndrome.

Once I had this diagnosis, I knew I had to work just one job. Too bad the job didn't last as long as I was hoping. Because I had to take time off from work to recuperate, I was placed on FMLA (Family Medical Leave Act). When I couldn't walk anymore, I was placed on restrictions which ended my job because my workplace couldn't accommodate. I was stunned. In less than four months, I had gone from two jobs to none. And it hurt. I didn't know my future. I applied for long-term disability and social security. I got it months later. Having no income for months was really difficult. I could barely survive. Thankfully, I was still living at home so I didn't have to worry about a roof over my head.

Midnight Demon

Intro To Psychiatrist

As you can see, I have had multiple therapies with a range of different kinds of therapists, from social workers to psychiatrists to psychologists. I have found that just having a degree doesn't make a good therapist. What matters is the connection you have with your patient. It is all part of the Aeschi model where you build a therapeutic relationship by just listening to the person's story without judgment or criticism, but with empathy and an understanding ear. I had a few of those but, unfortunately, they did not last…except for my current therapist. We have had our share of disagreements over the twelve years we have been together, but we worked through them like any good relationship does. From the start of my relationship with my psychiatrist, our alliance worked that way. She wasn't jamming pills down my throat or threatening me about my medication. It was my choice and she respected that. And I respected her.

I thought I would write about my psychiatrist as I seem to just focus on my therapists and it just doesn't seem right to exclude her. I met Dr. P. when I was seventeen. This year is our twentieth year working together. I read her story in a medical journal and I guess I was one of the few patients she decided to keep on. She wrote about how being a woman doctor in a man's profession was difficult, particularly in psychiatry. She also wrote about balancing work and motherhood. She spoke of her youngest having a hard time letting her go so she would stay by the door of her classroom to reassure her she was still there. That is the type of doctor I have. She has seen me at my worst, my best, and my saddest. Through every hospitalization and every bad day she has been there for me, always with that smile that makes me feel better. She has a way of talking to me and I know that tomorrow might be a better day because I know she is going to be there waiting for me to call, if need be. We both have this understanding that I cannot describe. We truly "get" each other and when we don't, we try to explain it so we *do* get it.

We have been through many medications. When I first saw her, I told her which medication I wanted to try. After all, I was proficient at reading the PDR (Physician's Desk Reference). Not too many people can decipher it. It was a big book with a lot of codes and references. But, at seventeen, I was able to get past the codes to get what I was looking for, which was usually the peaks and half-life of the drug. Half-life of a drug is when the drug, after a period of time, becomes inactive. I think I shocked her because I don't think any other teenager knew that. I wanted to be in the field in medicine and I still do. She told me that I could go to medical school and she meant it. To have her confident in me meant the world. That is what I love about her. She always believes in me when I can't believe in myself.

There was a time a few years ago when I was at my worst. I really was contemplating suicide and couldn't convey it to her so wrote her a goodbye email. This shocked her and I don't think I ever have seen her more scared of losing me. It kind of changed me. I don't write her these depressing emails as often anymore as I have my blog for that, but her hospitalizing me involuntarily changed our relationship for the better. I knew that if I ever was in need, she would take action. That was the only time she has had to do that in our twenty year relationship.

I still trust her with all my heart, but I hold back my suicidality from her at times. I still tell her I think about it. I just don't tell her my plans anymore for fear of hospitalization. The hospitalization was a strange time. I got things done at my job yet, at the same time, I was putting into motion a plan of killing myself. Luckily, the hospital helped put me on track and reset my thinking to other things.

We have built a solid foundation and it was because of the Aeschi model that was in place. If I

Midnight Demon

didn't have an open relationship with my psychiatrist, if I just had the standard fifteen minutes of seeing her for medication and that was all we talked about, I seriously doubt I would still be here today. Mostly, we talk about my ups and downs and how to get through them. We have exhausted the trials of medications so we are sticking with what we have right now. I don't know if I will ever be more stable on what drugs I am on right now versus the other twenty or so I have been on over the years. I have been on practically everything out there. SSRI's (selective serotonin reuptake inhibitors), e.g. Prozac; NSRI's (norepiphedrine/serotonin reuptake inhibitors), e.g. Cymbalta or duloxetine; tricyclics; mood stabilizers; lithium; anti-psychotics. I have probably been on everything at one time or another. The newer drugs have no hope for me because I have a sensitive stomach that makes me throw up after being on the medication for several months. I have been through that with the SSRI's. The only class of drugs I have not tried are the MAOI's or Mono-Amine Oxidaze Inhibitors. You have to be on a strict diet with this class of medication, and I love cheese and wine too much to give it up.

Since my first hospitalization at sixteen, I knew that I would have to take medication for my depression for the rest of my life. Depression is just like diabetes. Left untreated, it has disastrous consequences. Even after twenty years, I still have not found the right drug to make me happy or less depressed.

The road to finding the right combination of medication to treat my depression has been a long one. As I stated, I started taking psychotropic medication at sixteen. I started off with a tricyclic, nortryptaline. I found this medication to have a lot of side effects I didn't like. I started on it while I was in the hospital and continued it for a week. It takes several weeks for any antidepressant to take effect. Prozac was on the market, but I was too scared to try it. I moved through some of the tricyclics after this one, and after a few months, I stopped taking it because I found this class of drugs had no effect on me. I was also taking a phenothiazine, an antipsychotic, called Trilafon or perphenazine. This medication helped a lot with the voices that I have been hearing since I was five, but it made things really TOO quiet. I found I couldn't think while on this medication. My head was empty and I missed the voices so I stopped taking it. I now take Abilify (aripiprazole) to control the voices. I find that it helps me to think more clearly and I don't get paranoid as easily or get the ridiculous delusions I sometimes get.

When I was seventeen, I started Prozac. It was a new drug and I was afraid of it because, at the time, psychiatry was getting a bad name and being called "toxic", and pills were replacing psychotherapy. What the experts didn't quite know just ye, was that treatment and medication were key to a successful turnout.

I was placed on Prozac because I was desperate for relief of the darkness that invaded my soul. Within a few days, I was feeling much better. Around this time, I also came out of the closet with my homosexuality and this caused me to feel like a huge burden was lifted off my shoulders. For the first time in my life, I was happy. Maybe a little bit too happy.

A few weeks after starting Prozac, I had my first manic episode. I was not sleeping. I was not eating. I was feeling higher than a kite. It wasn't until I was at the train station and feeling invincible that I started to think maybe this drug was not to be continued. I felt like I could stop the train with my bare hands and that God had a special relationship with me. I called up Dr. P and we agreed to stop the medication. I was sad, but I knew that being too happy was not a good thing.

I was off medication a few weeks while the Prozac made its way out of my system. We thought that the mania was just drug-induced, but I was still having symptoms a month later so we started a trial of Lithium. At first, I didn't have any side effects. I hated getting my blood drawn for levels, but I thought maybe this was the right medication. As we increased the dose to get to the right blood

Midnight Demon

level, I started getting sick. I remember going to school after taking my dose. By the time I got to the second stop on the train, I was vomiting. There went that drug.

I then tried Tegretol, an anti-epileptic drug. I did fairly well on that for a few weeks. I had finally reached therapeutic blood levels when I got really sick. I broke out in a rash and was running a fever. I felt like hell, like the flu had hit me three hundred times harder than I ever experienced before. I called Dr. P. and she wanted me to have blood work done to make sure I wasn't developing one of the serious side effects, like Steven Johnson syndrome or aplastic anemia. It was found that I had an elevated white blood cell count and my ears were three times their normal size. I was miserable. Because I felt so weak, I asked if I could go to the local emergency room rather than go to Boston, where Dr. P practiced. It was there that I found out I had developed an infection, in addition to having an allergic reaction to the Tegretol. This left me so bummed and I hated taking drugs after that, which made Dr. P. nervous. She didn't want me to try anything else. It took several months to even think of trying another trial of medication again. Both of us were weary of it.

Eventually, my depression got worse and I needed something to take the edge off. Back to the trials. We started with something slow…Zoloft. I did well on this medication for a few years. However, even at the maximum dosage, it stopped working for me. I then started to get the dry heaves. It wasn't until I realized that the peak of this medication always coincided with my getting sick did I put two and two together. From there, we went to Celexa, Paxil, Doxepin, but either they didn't provide me with great relief or they had to be discontinued due to side effects. I really hated the Paxil because it caused me to gain weight. I tried the atypical Amoxetine and had no success with it. I was placed on another mood stabilizer, valproic acid/Depakote, but I hated the blood draws so I stopped it. Nothing seemed to work for me or, if it did, it stopped working after a year or two. This depression was harder to battle than I imagined and my suicidality was always a threat.

It wasn't until I was in the throes of yet another crippling depression that Dr. P. had the startling revelation of trying me on oxcarbazepine (Trileptal). I have found success with this. I have been on this for the past several years and it seems to help. I finally found something that worked. Even though it didn't cure me of my depression, it helped lessen the symptoms and kept the mood swings in check. During this trial, I also was placed on Cymbalta, the latest SNRI out on the market that was supposed to help with the pain of depression, but it didn't help me at all. It might have helped me in the first few months, but it lost its effectiveness. And like previous SSRI's, it made me sick. I had waited for years for it to come on the market because I had done so well on its precursor, Remeron. Remeron worked really well for me, but its effectiveness was limited to only thirty days. That was it.

Cymbalta promised to help and it was the last drug in the arsenal. It turned out to be another loser. I couldn't tolerate the dry heaves that I got from these antidepressants. I was deeply frustrated that I was doing what the books had said, that medication and therapy were key, but I couldn't find a medication that worked for me. I am thankful that starting the oxcarbazepine did work for me. I really noticed a difference with this medication within a few weeks of starting it. It really saved my life.

Midnight Demon

Where I Am Meant To Be

There was a point in time about five years ago where the American Association of Suicidology was coming to Boston for their annual conference. I wanted to go so I submitted a paper for their poster session. To my disbelief, I got accepted! I was still working as an undergraduate at UMass/Boston, and I got accepted for this prestigious organization. I couldn't believe it! For that week, it was the happiest I had ever been. I really found what my purpose was in life…to become more of a geek and join these professionals. The poster session was really awesome. I had a lot of people comment on it. My psychiatrist was all excited and wanted to come, but something came up and she couldn't attend. My therapist did come and she witnessed Dr. David Jobes shaking my hand. I was a nervous wreck. I swear I could have died after that. I was never as excited as I was that night. I met another grad student, Lily, and we are still good friends. We keep in touch after all this time and I still want to visit her in Lubbock, Texas, but time and finances always gets in the way.

What I took away from this conference was a huge appreciation for the work these professionals do. I had a pre-conference workshop with Dr. Jobes for the CAMS model and it was great. Collaborating, Assessment, and Managing of Suicidality, is a framework in which the clinician and client collaborate on treatment goals for dealing with suicidal thoughts. I learned how to administer it and took away from it that I could use this from the point of view of both a patient and therapist. The SSF (suicide status form) was the icing on the cake. Learning how to administer this important assessment tool is crucial in assessing a suicidal person's risk and state of mind. These forms assess the suicide risk and also the factors that are pressuring the suicidal ideation. The forms are Initial, Tracking, and Outcome.

What was really amazing was that my therapist showed up to this presentation. I really appreciated her support as I was so nervous that these clinicians would find out I was a patient and have me hospitalized. It was a crazy thought, but I still was thinking of killing myself, even though this conference gave me a new purpose in life.

My second conference did not go as well as the first one. I was haggard from the travel to Baltimore and didn't take away anything other than that I was a hopeless case that no one would want. I even talked to the director of the Mayo Clinic and told him my symptoms and he just was so flustered he didn't know what to tell me on how to deal with that. I felt really hopeless about my future and all I wanted to do was leave. I didn't meet up with my friends from the previous conference and just caught the earlier train back to Boston. That trip left me so downhearted. The whole way back, I cried and wrote about how I felt.

I did get autographs from my favorite writers, including Jobes (again), Mark Goldblatt, and Terry Maltsberger. Dr. Maltsberger is one of Boston's most famous psychiatrists in the field of suicide. It was great to hear him at the pre-conference workshop that I attended. Jobes was not there that day, but there were others that were focused on the Aeschi model. What I took from the conference was what stuff I already knew… that knowing the patient's story is crucial in learning why the patient wants to kill him or herself. That is what the suicidal wants. They just want to be heard.

Midnight Demon

Blog Post About Aeschi

While I was at Starbucks the other day, I was taking notes on my Aeschi book, Building a Therapeutic Alliance with Suicidal Patients. I was writing down what I had highlighted, but there was too much information that I didn't highlight that I needed to share so I gave up on it…for now. This book is so powerful that you really need time and energy not only to read it, but to digest its contents. It guides you to what the model is and how to go about being a better therapist to handle a suicidal person. It provides empirical support as well as experience. The provider needs to change to a more patient-oriented model in dealing with suicidal patients.

The suicidal patient just wants to be heard, to have a voice. Most suicidal people think they are too hopeless to think that talking with someone will help them, but if you are one of these people, I know that by reading this you are trying to find the answers you need to not commit suicide.

I wanted to write about the Aeschi model and also how Dr. Jobes came into my life through his work. I really believe that if more clinicians took this approach and used Jobes' assessment tool, the SSF (suicide status form), and his framework for CAMS to treat their suicidal patients, or at least have this approach in inpatient settings, there might be less suicide.

The road to finding the answers to help yourself is long. But when you are contemplating suicide, there is not a whole lot out there. Through my research about psychological pain, I found that Edwin Shneidman, Ronald Holden, and David Jobes helped me find the answers I was looking for and helped me to augment the therapeutic bond with my therapist. Through CAMS and finding the Aeschi model, I knew that I was onto something.

CAMS evolved into a clinical need to assess, evaluate, track the outcome of, and find out the risk factors of suicidality. Today this assessment has used the SSF, Suicide Status Form, to do all these things while providing compassionate care.

CAMS was conceived to assess suicide risk, as well as to develop a suicide specific treatment. Because initial intakes sometimes get lost in the system, Dr. Jobes wanted a way to track the outcome of suicidal cases so that there would be better adherence to someone who was suicidal. By developing the CAMS method over the course of twenty-five years, he had done just that. Now, people who are suicidal don't get lost in the system. There are many reasons why people leave treatment, but not understanding that someone was suicidal was a big one. In the SSF, there is a space on the form that asks whether the patient has terminated, gone to the hospital, or has a follow up appointment. (See Jobes, Managing Suicidal Risk, 2006 for more information)

Midnight Demon

The Aeschi Model

The Aeschi Model (pronounced Eshi) is a patient-oriented model, meaning that the patient has more of a say over treatment than the clinician does. It takes away the clinician as the expert. What has been found is that the provider-oriented model doesn't work as patients can get frustrated over the "provider knows best" thinking. The patient is not being heard and retreats from treatment. The Aeschi works toward a collaborative effort with the patient and provider working together to find out what is at the heart of the suicidality.

The gist of the Aeschi philosophy is to have the suicidal person be in charge of treatment and have a voice, a novel idea when so many clinicians think they know better than the patient and, therefore, take charge of their treatment, with the patient not having a say. I know that if my therapist had been in this category, I probably would not be here. I believe that if there is a collaborative effort between the therapist and patient, there will be a higher success rate than if the therapist has the one track mind of he/she knows best. But the nice thing is that the Aeschi Model doesn't have to focus on one discipline. It can work for social workers, psychologists, psychiatrists, mental health workers, etc. It just takes a little courage to step out of the normal boundaries and put the patient first, to let the patient tell their story without being judgmental or critical. After the patient tells their story, there is an openness. Once the clinician has a sympathetic and empathic ear that is open to whatever the patient is saying, the real journey begins.

This model is the new age of what therapy should be. I know that if I didn't develop this kind of relationship with my therapist, I probably wouldn't be here. I once had a therapist that was trying to cram dialectical behavioral therapy down my throat, saying it was the answer to my problem. I didn't believe it for one second. One of the exercises had you think and write down all your negative thoughts for the day. At the end of the day, I had over a hundred thoughts of wanting to hurt/kill myself. I felt like an asshole. How was this treatment supposed to help me feel better when I felt worse? I know of some success stories with this treatment, but it just wasn't for me. I'd rather go along with the story model, to tell my story to my therapist and see what we can make out of it to help me. I no longer see this therapist.

    I now have an eclectic therapist that I am trying to teach suicidology to. She has learned the terminology fairly well. When I am in suicidal crisis, she runs down the press, perturbation, and psychache. These three things are what Dr. Shneidman calls the "Suicidal Model". If these three things reach a 5-5-5 on a scale of 1-5, suicide is imminent. Unbearable pain cannot last more than a few days time before being acted upon. Bringing down the press, the pressure of built up emotions can lower a suicide risk, as well as lowering the perturbation (the feeling of needing to get something done now). Psychache is a little harder to lower, but I have found that having an understanding ear that is open to my thoughts of darkness, no matter how truly dark they get, is what helps lower my pain.

    This year is my twentieth year with my psychiatrist. From the beginning, I knew she was different than any other doctor I ever met. She listens to me. She helped me take charge of my treatment. She didn't tell me that this medication should be jammed down my throat in order to help. In fact, it was the opposite. I was telling her what medications I wanted to be on. No doctor does that, except for one that has a level of trust. She follows the Aeschi model, even before the concept was formally developed and expressed in a book. There have been many hospitalizations, many trying times with me over the years, but she was always there to lend a sympathetic ear. She always believed in me when I didn't believe in myself.

Midnight Demon

Aeschi

When did I first get involved in this model? It was in 2010 and I was in the midst of another suicidal episode. I wanted to kill myself before Thanksgiving. But then Jobes came out with his book and it took me a week of reading it to come to terms with my suicidality and put my suicidal feelings on hold. I really thought they had the very best book out there for clinicians, who wanted to deal with suicidal clients, to read. If you are not dealing with someone who is suicidal, this book is pretty useless.

What I got from this book was something I never experienced before. I felt like they knew what was in my head. These clinicians that I have never worked with or seen before brought to life what I was thinking while I was reading it. In the final chapter, it says that this work cannot be applied because clinicians still rely on their own interviewing techniques to assess suicide risk, and it's true. The adage "you cannot teach an old dog new tricks" cannot be said of suicide training. You must learn the new tricks if you truly want to save a life. I recently asked my psychiatrist if she would use CAMS for a suicidal client and her answer was not shocking in that she didn't know if she would or not. I guess it depends on the circumstances. If you have someone that doesn't have a good understanding of the English language or is illiterate, it might pose a problem. Or if the person speaks another language other than English, it will definitely be a barrier. Another disadvantage would be to those that are not competent due to severe mental retardation or disability. I can understand those cases. But they need to know their clients. It might be scary introducing this model to your client, but it might also save their life. So the choice is to go the route you know or change. And isn't that what therapy is all about?

It always surprises me the way people think about suicide and suicidal thinking. They think that you must be angry at someone or something. That something is keeping you here or you would have done it, or that you are all talk until you do it. Or that you have to be in some tremendous pain to think of such things. I guess there are still some people that think because they have had some experience with suicide, because they themselves have thought about or even acted on it, that they are experts. Well, they are, to a degree. Not all people want to help after they have attempted it. Some shy away from it and call it just a bad experience, vowing never to go down that road again. Some continue to be suicidal, like myself. But I still want to help those that are suffering because it means that someone cares.

      I have been writing for months (or what seems like months) about having a suicidal plan. The only people that know are my readers and my therapist. I am afraid of bringing up the subject with my psychiatrist for fear of being hospitalized against my will. There are days, like today, that I don't think I will go through with my plan. Then there are times that I think I will, just for kicks and giggles. But the hardest part of this crazy plan is that it is not too detailed. I have a vague idea about what I will be doing to kill myself. And because of this vagueness, I feel that I shouldn't go through with it. The last thing I want is another failed attempt. That would devastate me more than anything.

Midnight Demon

Early Life

I don't like to talk about my early life. It is too painful and involves nightmares and flashbacks. I grew up in a chaotic home; however, if you were to ask my mother, I grew up "pleasantly". Denial was a big thing in our house. We couldn't be ourselves. At an early age, I learned that I wanted out of my family. I even contemplated joining the Navy to get away. I figured I loved the ocean and ships so what better career?

All of that came to a screeching halt when I was diagnosed with major depression with psychotic tendencies at sixteen. My career in the military was over before it had even begun. I was devastated. I had heard voices since I was five-years-old. They started off as voices that I heard from the TV that followed me around. Then, as I grew up, the voices stayed and I had someone to converse with in the dead of night. I didn't think anything was wrong with this as long as my parents didn't know. Sometimes when I was agitated, it would appear that I was talking to myself but, in reality, I was really talking to the voices.

My father was a mean bastard, though he was a nice guy to others. He loved to torment my sisters and me through physical and psychological abuse. My mother didn't do much about it.

I lived in a small town, a suburb of Boston. Though the population has now increased as they have built up, the place is pretty much the same. Most of the Italians have moved out, and other ethnic groups have moved in. I graduated with a class of 150 students. I started my freshman year with 250. Not too many of the kids I grew up with stayed in college. I grew up at a time where drugs and teen pregnancy were huge factors in drop out rates. My middle sister did not graduate from high school after we moved to another larger city my junior year. Moving was tough as I loved the house, but not the memories. We moved to a quiet neighborhood on a dead end street, and I found the quietness of the street disturbing. Within the first three months of living there, I had three panic attacks. I got paranoid. I ended up in the hospital for the third and fourth time. Suicide was all I could think about. I had to get away and if I couldn't get away in the military, I wanted to die. The voices helped me to see that I was a worthless nothing that didn't deserve to live. Medication controlled the voices, but I didn't feel right afterwards. I felt alone. I couldn't think. I couldn't even hear my own thoughts.

    I stopped taking the medication and the "bad" voices went away. I still had the trials and tribulations of antidepressant medications. Nothing worked for me, or if it did, not for long. Prozac, which really helped me to get out of the hole I was in, caused me to have a manic episode. I was then placed on many mood stabilizers to quiet down this side of me that I didn't know existed. I thought I just had depression, but it turned out I also had Bipolar II Disorder. It is a disorder where I have infrequent hypomanic episodes. It is treated the same way as with any other bipolar disorder…mood stabilizers and antidepressants. And as I also get psychotic, I take an antipsychotic. Since most of the antidepressants stop working for me or make me sick, I have mostly been on a mood stabilizer and antipsychotic. This combination seems to help, but I still get the dark moods, the suicidal thoughts, the severe hopelessness, and anguish that causes me to think that ending my life is the only way out.

Midnight Demon

Mentioning Of Suicide, Therapist Panics

I had been seeing an interim therapist while waiting to go to college after I graduated high school. I was seeing someone in the local mental health center and I was supposed to see her for the summer because my current therapist got laid off due to budget cuts.

Somewhere in the middle of that summer, about three weeks before I was supposed to leave for college, I reached the lowest point in my life. Like anyone else would do, I told my therapist that I was having suicidal feelings. She then did something totally unexpected. She took a deep breath, held it, let it go, then sat there stunned. She didn't know what to do. She asked if I needed to be seen by someone in the emergency room and I forget what I said. I think I said I did because I went to the local hospital and was admitted for two weeks. I was glad my summer job had come to a close so I didn't have to worry about work.

What I didn't realize was that suicide is a big deal in the mental health field. The therapist didn't want to take me back after my admission so I was stuck seeing a resident, who basically said it was her or the hospital. I didn't have a choice of people to talk to. Sure, they were fine in the confined settings of a hospital, but they were taboo in an outpatient setting. I always knew it was high risk, but it wasn't until I entered into the field of suicidology that I really understand what it meant to be suicidal…not just as a patient, but also as a clinician. I am not a clinician, but I do have a clinical way of thinking about things. I might not be trained, but I have more experience in therapy than a new graduate or even someone who has spent their lifetime doing this. I like to think of myself as an expert but, then again, all people who have attempted suicide feel that they are.

What struck me was the legality of the dreaded no-suicide contracts, the risk for malpractice, the ethical responsibility of the patient in the course of therapy, and the risk of losing the patient. Those are some pretty big reasons NOT to take on a client, but what if you were in the situation that I was in? I already had an "established" therapist who got cold feet when I told her I was thinking about killing myself. And in the age of the internet, I find that I am not the only one who has had this experience.

    I also have had trouble finding another therapist. My current therapist, though she still gets anxious when I talk about suicide, is thirty miles from me and I don't have a car. We communicate solely by phone, unless I can take my sister's car every so often to drive the forty-five minutes to hour drive both ways. I have tried to find a therapist within a five mile radius of my house and have failed not once, not twice, not three times, but ten fucking times!!! That is right. I called ten different therapists and they all turned me down because I had a history of being suicidal. It hurts and sucks. They just asked the question, I answered honestly, and got either referred to another therapist or was turned down outright.

    During the course of trying to find a therapist, I got hospitalized. I could finally see a therapist face-to-face, but when I did, he was scared of me. Beads of sweat were coming down his face and he had a high-pitched, nervous laugh. I could tell he did not want to treat me. He didn't want to lose me because I was such high-risk. What makes you high risk? Having a significant history of suicide attempts; a history of being abused either physically, emotionally, sexually, or all three; constant suicidal thoughts; and feeling hopeless. There are other criteria, but those jump out at me as the most significant. I once went to a suicidology conference where I listed the prominent symptoms of my condition and had it reviewed by one of the suicidologists. He didn't want to touch me with a ten foot pole. I never felt so hopeless in my life. At that point, I knew there was no hope for me, and that I was destined to always be suicidal, or at least have suicidal thoughts. But it shocked me that this expert had no advice for me other than saying good luck.

    To be a suicidal patient and have nowhere to go is a tough situation. You depend on the therapist to be there for you and to talk openly about any topic you want to talk about, including suicide. But what do you do when the therapist has no clue? You would think that the therapist would know how to handle the situation. You are, after all, trusting this person to give you advice about your life. It seems kind of late to start the training while you are in crisis. It's not like you can put your life on hold while the therapist gets a clue. All I can say is to be patient. Don't buy into a no suicide contract because they don't work.

    Go to the American Association of Suicidology's website to help both you and your therapist. There are not too many therapists that know how to handle suicidal crises, and each state has its own rules regarding suicidal safety. The best advice I can offer is for you both be honest with one another and to listen to each other to weather out the storm. Have a safety plan in place. Use a crisis response plan. Pick up the book, Managing Suicidal Risk by David Jobes and give it to your therapist. If the therapist says she or he cannot work with you anymore, find someone who can. That might take some doing and some time, but you WILL find someone that is not afraid of suicide.

Midnight Demon

Gender Identity

I have been thinking about what led up to my suicide attempt and, frankly, it's hard to determine now that so many years have passed. I know that I was in terrible psychological pain and I wanted to die. Up until then, I really had not tried to seriously kill myself, but I knew the pills I had would do the job, even if it would take some time.

My family was not supportive. They thought they were, but they actually made things worse. During one of my hospitalizations prior to the attempt, I remember my mother wanted the psychiatrist to put me under hypnosis as a cathartic measure to get all my problems out at once. She didn't realize that it would take time and that it might actually harm me. I knew it was a crazy notion and I was upset that she confronted the staff with these demands. I eventually prohibited her from coming to the unit as it was too upsetting for me to see her so hurt. She wanted me to have a close relationship with her, but after she abandoned me after my first attempt when I was ten, I lost confidence in her ability as a mother. I just knew that she would not be the one to go to when I was really upset. I felt like such a burden to her. I felt like she loved my sisters more than she loved me. We never got along. She never had to scold me because I always listened and was a "good girl". It pained me every single time someone told me this.

I didn't put my transgender issues and being depressed/suicidal together until I was in my thirties. I always knew that, one day, I would just grow into a man until. I eventually realized that was not going to happen unless I started with hormones. I never voiced this to my mother, especially after how she reacted to my homosexuality. I knew there was no way for her to process her first born being a son rather than a daughter. But even as I am writing this, it is difficult to process.

I first realized I was different when I was in kindergarten. I noticed the other girls liked playing make-up and played with dolls, while I played with the trucks and other boy toys. My best friend all through childhood was a boy and I wanted to be just like him. Then I realized there were changes around the age of eight. I started developing and I had no idea why I was so damn sad. I started having a chest and had to wear things called bras. It was just too much for me. I began to shut down. I was so depressed, but I felt like I couldn't talk to anyone around me about it for fear of being called crazy.

    Around the time I began menstruating was the worst. I prayed for death. I was really down and I couldn't understand what was happening. I had thoughts of being a man, yet my body was reacting like a female. It didn't make sense to me. I really had no idea what was happening. I acted like a tomboy and every one assumed I would grow out of it…until I started buying men's clothing. I just liked them more than women's and they made me feel more comfortable. I knew what my size was because it made sense to me more than women's clothes. But my sisters and mother didn't understand. I am not sure what my father thought of my dress because I could care less. I now have minimal contact with him since he fell off the pedestal I put him on years ago.

    During my teenage years, I found out that my father was a cheater and a pathological liar. My mother confronted him one night and he lied and said that he would never cheat on her. I found out that while he was working with a woman for the social center, he asked her out several times. It was then that I found out my father often danced with women. This would explain why he came home as late as four in the morning. He would always lie and say he was playing cards, but it was not true. How could he be playing cards and dancing at the same time??

    He was not the best father. He was a very selfish man who only thought about his needs. He had always been that way. Although now he has taken to my little sister and doesn't think of his two other children. But then again, my middle sister and I don't like having contact with him anyway. It is our choice. We will talk to him when he comes over to my sister's house, but other than that, I will not talk

Midnight Demon

to him. He just aggravates the crap out me with his vengeful attitude. I know I have his disposition. I can get hot-tempered like he does, but I learned many years ago not be selfish and to always give before receiving. I guess that is why it is so hard to get things for myself and to have self-care because I view this as being selfish.

At the age of fifteen, I realized that I needed help. That I was not right. That things in the house were not right. I didn't know that part of the reason I was so miserable was because of my issues with my gender identity. If I realized that sooner, things might be different today and maybe I wouldn't have tried to kill myself so many times over the years.

In my teenage years, cutting provided me comfort. But it was difficult to hide because I liked wearing short-sleeved shirts. I couldn't wear long-sleeved shirts and even if I did, I usually rolled the sleeves up, exposing my injured wrist/arm. I once kept a wound open for a month. I just kept cutting it every day as a release of the pain that I was feeling. Each time, I cut deeper and deeper hoping to do damage, but it never got that far.

After two months of cutting, it lost its appeal for me. I was seeing Marilyn at this time and she was into Dialectical Behavioral Therapy (DBT). One of the rules of this therapy is no therapeutic contact 24 hours after a self-harm incident. It drove me crazy. I think it was to change the behavior, but it never did. I stopped doing it because it just lost its usefulness.

I think it was at this time that I decided to experiment by overdosing. I would take, say, ten tablets at time and see what happened. I remember I had taken something like thirty-two milligrams of my antipsychotic medication to see if I could get relief of psychological pain. All it did was make me very groggy and messed with my fine motor skills, such as writing. I developed shaky hands while trying to write.

Midnight Demon

Mourning Loss Of Self

    I was reading my support group email and a friend was telling the group how you need to mourn the loss of your old self because you are never going to get back to it. Then a fellow blogger wrote the same sentiments about her illness and how disabled she felt, but didn't realize how much of herself had gone by the wayside since becoming ill. She was crying as a way to mourn that loss. It got me thinking…maybe I am so suicidal because my grief is just too great.

    I got CES at the age of twenty-five, and in the past year-and-a-half, I have been diagnosed with a nerve condition called Complex Regional Pain Syndrome (CRPS), which is the chief source of my foot/ankle/leg pain. It was caused by already damaged nerves. Aren't I the lucky one to get both conditions? Since my diagnoses, I have been really depressed. I know there is no treatment other than opioid therapy. Though I have been in therapy with the same therapist for the last twelve-and-a-half years, I still have not thought about how much these conditions have affected my life until now. I can no longer work. At one time in my life, I was working three jobs. Now I can barely do one. Before going on disability, I was working two, but I wasn't happy. Both jobs were stressful and caused me some sleepless nights.

    But then I sprained my ankle and everything started to go downhill. I couldn't figure out why the ankle, which should have healed in the allotted time, was still causing me pain; why my leg still had swelling; why my foot and ankle were swollen. It didn't make any sense. I saw one doctor after another. Podiatrists, orthopedists, physiatrists, neurologists. None could give me a clue, until the symptoms became worse and a picture of CRPS started to emerge.

    By that time, I was having difficulty working both jobs. I ended up going to the emergency room in severe pain, pain that was causing me to think of suicide as a solution to end it. I went to physical therapy and they were the ones to notice I wasn't walking correctly. My foot pulls at muscles it's not

Midnight Demon

supposed to while I walk, but only does so when I become fatigued. Which, one physical therapist showed, happens very quickly because I never regained my strength in my foot after getting CES. I never thought that I would be disabled at the age of 36. And it hurts. Not having the social support of my co-workers anymore hurts. Not having contact with people outside of my family hurts. My friends that I thought would always be there are there no longer.

    I guess when I had uncontrollable sobbing episodes it was because of my grief that I have been avoiding all this time. I didn't know how to deal with it. I never thought that I would be in mourning. I never thought that I would lose my job because I couldn't walk anymore. I *am* able to walk, just not for long distances. I can't stand for more than twenty minutes without pain. I used to be able to do so much and now I can't do anything.

    And, because I am not financially stable, I can't even go back to college while I ponder my next move. College is too expensive for me to afford, even at the state college. I know I could put some time into getting a grant or something, but I wonder if I am too "old" to get it. I had to put my college education on hold because of my mental illness back in 2008 and I have not returned since. I am not sure I could walk around campus and do the stairs like I used to anyway. There is a lot of loss in my life on a very personal level. How do you mourn the loss of your functions, as well? How do you get used to not doing something as simple as walking? I have had to relearn to walk again twice in my life. How many people can say that?

    It makes me angry at times. I guess that is why I have been having fits of anger for no reason. I will just be in my room playing on my laptop or writing when, all of a sudden, waves of anger will wash over me. I guess it is all part of the grieving process. Isn't one of them denial?

Blog Post: Loss Of Self

The stages of grief are denial, isolation, anger, bargaining, depression, and acceptance.

I broached the subject of grief with my therapist. She hasn't received her packet of letters that describes my grief and how I think I should address it. I couldn't bring myself to tell her that I think the reason for my craziness the last few months has to do with not dealing with my grief. Of course, I didn't think much of it until I asked if grief can cause psychosis. Then I just shut down. Thank god it was the end of session. She wanted to see me the next day, but I told her Tuesday was fine. It will give me more time to think about how to approach this.

She encouraged me to write about this stuff, but I don't know how. Just thinking about my losses makes me extremely sad. It's like knocking the wind out of me. I mean, I used to be able to work two jobs and now I can't even work one. I was stable enough to work in one job for fourteen years, and then my foot got messed up. I don't know if I could work at the same job again. I would like to, but I can't be running around like I used to. The things is, being a lab assistant, you sometimes have to do phlebotomy (draw blood) and I was never keen on that.

It still hurts that after fourteen years of service, I was not accommodated by my job. I never told anyone how bad losing my job was. It also sucks that I can't do my other job of driving around Boston picking up samples because my driving record got messed up. I got a speeding ticket one morning because I was too sleepy to notice I was over the speed limit. Then, because I couldn't pay the fine, my license got suspended. It took me almost a year to get it all cleared up. But it is going to take a while for me to have a "good" driving record again. And that kills me. I know it doesn't matter now

Midnight Demon

because by the time I have a car of my own, my record will be clean.

    I really have other deep losses such as the loss of myself and the loss of my abilities. Walking used to be my joy. I was able to walk long distances and think nothing of it. It never bothered me. Sometimes it did when I used to get cramps if I walked too far and didn't drink enough water. But other than that, I really enjoyed walking to the train station, which is about a mile away. I used to do the Walk for Hunger, which is a twenty mile walk around Boston. I haven't done that in years, but I am determined to do it again one year, as long as I go slowly. I will have to do a lot of training to work up to it because, right now, my limit is four blocks.

    Then I have the loss of my bodily functions. I never thought that, at the age of thirty-six, I would have to wear diapers to events that last longer than a few hours. This is because I no longer get the signals to my brain that my bladder is full. Once I am full, I start leaking until I go. It isn't until I feel wet that I ask myself the last time I went. Bowel movements are a different story. If you are the squeamish type, I would stop reading right now because this could be disgusting to you.

    If my stools are soft, I don't feel them as they move out. If I have the runs, I can quickly have an accident as I can't hold them long, although I have been lucky the last few times holding them in by not letting my farts loose. If I lose control of my farts, I lose control of my stool and…well, you know. It has only happened to me a few times. The worst was when I took too many fiber pills and thought I was farting, but I was really shitting myself. That was a lesson learned. I usually take Senna because I find that it is the only thing that makes me go without too much trouble. Too much, however, can cause very bad cramps and possible accidents. Every time I have an accident or have skid marks because I didn't wipe myself well enough, I lose it. I really go into a darker place and usually want to kill myself. The same with when I have a urine accident, but I am getting used to them. Having stool in my pants is a real downer, though. I don't think anyone can get used to that. It makes you feel so small. And people take it for granted that their bodies will tell them these things. My body, because of the nerve damage, no longer does. And it is a HUGE loss. Again, not something I wanted to deal with.

Then, of course, there is the loss of where I should be now had my mental illness not shut me down and forced me to stop college. I call this the "if only's". If only I didn't have a psychotic breakdown in 2008, how different would my life have been? If only I went to a four year school instead of getting just my Associate's Degree, would I be better off now than I was back then? If only I had decided to work part-time and go to college full-time, would I have been better mentally than I am now? Would the financial strain of not working have been too much? Would the strain of going to college full-time have been my downfall? I can't change any of it, but not being able to go back is a huge loss to me. I should have just made a simple phone call to put my loans into deferment and I would have been able to go back. Now I am just sitting on my ass doing nothing most days. I think me not going to back to college is the most painful because I loved my studies. It didn't matter what they were. I just loved being in academia. Psychology is really my thing, and I know I could have been a good therapist. But I don't think those dreams are ever going to come true.

Then you take into account all the times I have been suicidal. It is a loss because I am still having to piece my life back together and I don't like it. I'd rather be pushing up daisies for eternity. But as past blogs have talked about, I can't kill myself any more than I can make a gourmet dinner, but it hurts to go on living like this.

I'm wondering if going through the stages of grief will help my mental state at all. I have been in denial for so long that I don't know if I can really go through it. But I know it will be an interesting topic for my therapist, if I ever show her my writings and she actually reads them.

I'm reading Noonday Demon and it is reminding me that depression is a passing illness. What you feel today, you won't feel tomorrow. I find this true.

Blog Post: Façades Sept 23, 2013

    I guess I am a coward for not going ahead with the plans. And it sucks now that I have to live with this. I can't die and I am not living. How to keep going? That is the problem and it makes me so sad.

    I saw my PCP yesterday and, to him, I appeared cheerful. Oh, how I deceive people. I am so used to hiding what I feel that I guess I have the knack of deception. The day before, I was in the throes of horrendous pain, and yesterday I was cheerful. Funny, I didn't feel cheerful. My head was filled with suicidal thoughts so how could I be cheerful? I guess the most depressed person is the best hidden. I have always been able to hide my pain, even as he was poking around my injured foot. I don't know if he realizes the struggle I go through every day. No one does. Maybe I should look into other methods of self-destruction, but I doubt I can go through with it so what is the point of thinking of another plan?

    I often wonder what would happen in the aftermath of my death. Would I be missed? I often write a suicide note saying no one is to blame. The only person to really blame is myself. IF I had only done things differently…I'm not sure what…maybe I wouldn't want to end my life. I just know that writing about it is the only escape I have left. No one wants to hear about how suicidal I am anymore. I am sure my therapist would rejoice if I never mentioned suicide again. Maybe if I wasn't so open with these suicidal thoughts, they would go away. This is something I have contemplated for a while now. But the nitwit assesses my psychache most sessions so I cannot lie or betray her confidence in me. If I say "No, I have no thoughts", I doubt she will believe me anyway.

    Every day for the past several years, I've thought about ending my life. Some days, I think about it more than others. Sometimes pain dictates the severity of killing myself and the need to escape from it. That is all I desire…an escape from consciousness. Escape is the biggest reason for suicide. Escape from intolerable feelings of

Midnight Demon

distress one constantly feels. In my case, I want to escape from the emotional and physical pain of living. It's gotten to the point that I can no longer distinguish between the two when taking a psychological pain scale assessment.

I just wish the pain would stop. No one can find a way to relieve it. Icing/elevating/resting for the past year have not helped. It is very debilitating to be in pain, yet it can't be relieved by ordinary measures. And the worst part is being passed around from doctor to doctor. It's the merry-go-round of health care. This doctor says it's this and refers you to another doctor, who refers you to yet another doctor where the answers are the same. Nothing is wrong with you that they can fix so it has to be coming from the back, but even the neurosurgeon says there is nothing wrong. So why bother going to all these doctors anymore?

While visiting my primary, he wanted me to go back to my physiatrist (doctor that specializes in muscles and joints). I am done seeing specialists. Besides this doctor moved her office to another site that I can't get to. I don't believe there is public transportation to her new office. I really liked her, too. She has been the most straight forward of all the other doctors I have seen. And besides, I know she is just going to say I have tendonitis. A tendonitis that flares up unexpectedly when I am at rest? Makes no sense. But then she'll go back to the diagnosis of Complex Regional Pain Syndrome, and I'll be sent back to my primary for pain management. And so the flip-flop goes.

Yesterday, I had some weird symptoms that I believe are from the anti-psychotic that I take to control my voices. It was like I was having Parkinson's symptoms. When I came home last night, it wasn't so bad. I didn't take my regular dose and took some Ativan to calm me down as it was making me anxious. I emailed my psychiatrist to let her know and I still have not heard back from her. I see her on Friday anyways and, other than me skipping and lowering my dose, there is nothing more that she can do. The only thing that sucks after this is that my hands feel fatigued.

I had a good night last night and I went out to dinner with some friends, but a Facebook status that I posted a few days ago came back to haunt me. I wrote something to the effect that no one cares that I am in pain and that I am not doing anything for anyone anymore. It really pissed me off that, weeks afterwards, I was still getting reminded of that post. I don't understand why people take things so seriously, then can't let it go. Isn't it obvious I was having a bad night? Couldn't you just say you were sorry I was having a rough time? But no, the part about me saying that no one cares is the foremost thing that should be talked about.

This is what I posted -- "Everyone turns a blind eye to the pain I experience every day. So be it. When they ask for something, I will just tell them I can't do it because of pain. Maybe then they will get the message. I am too tired of fighting. All my thoughts are dark and no one cares or gives a shit".

I don't think I offended anyone or singled out any one person but, apparently, I was not supposed to feel this way and post it. I will post what I want to post. Just like I will post whatever I feel with my blogs. The sad part is that a couple of close friends reacted to the status, but not one family member did. Shows that you don't have to be a relative to care.

I don't remember this post. It was written while I was "Mr. Hyde". I get into these frames of mind where I become another person. I might have a little of Dissociative Identity Disorder (formerly known as Multiple Personality Disorder). What I have noticed when I am in these states is that I am not "aware" of myself like I am when I am less depressed. I am usually highly suicidal and all I think about is ending my life. I will make plans, which have mostly consisted of writing goodbye letters to people I care about. In my last state, I wrote to my friend in South Africa and I wished him well. I told him I loved him and that the struggle was too much for me to bear. The next morning, I had no recollection of what I did. I woke up in a "good" mood and was surprised to receive a message from my friend saying that he was really worried about me. I

Midnight Demon

had no clue why. It was like I had blacked out, except that I don't drink. These mood shifts worry me because, although I have not done anything, I fear that I will snap and will act on my feelings one day. Also, when I am in this frame of mind, I do not want to talk to anyone so using the crisis response plan that my therapist has in place is useless. My thoughts are centered around ending my life and putting things in place so that I can kill myself. I have noticed that it seems to happen when I am extremely fatigued, in a lot of physical pain, and can't get to sleep. I usually call this state "The Midnight Demons" because it is like a demonic possession comes over me until I pass out.

I also remember feeling a lot of psychological pain. It becomes very intense. Looking back the next day, I really don't like being in this state. I am trying to find ways of grounding myself, but I have not been too successful at it. So I try and make sure not to get too fatigued and control my physical pain the best I can. I also notice that the voices become louder and will have conversations with me late at night. This prevents me from actually lying down and sleeping no matter how physically tired I am. It's worse than having the "brain won't shut off" feeling. Of course, if people continue to talk and ask questions to you most of the night, you will find yourself getting agitated and not being able to sleep. What's worse is that you fight the medication causing you to fall asleep. It's not a good thing.

The earliest time I remember these dissociative states happening to me was back in 2009 when I was under a lot of stress and pressure with my job. I had decided to write to my psychiatrist, who knew me very well, that I couldn't go on. I wish I had a copy of that letter now to show you how distraught I was and that she had good reason for hospitalizing me. It was so depressing. But I wrote another one, though still in the frame of mind that I was. It was a longer version, which thanks her for doing the best she could for me. When she called me the next morning and couldn't get in touch with me, she Section 12'd me. Section 12 is the Massachusetts statute that allows mental health professionals the right to involuntarily hospitalize someone in danger of harming themselves or others. Police and paramedics were sent to my home. I have never before felt like an idiot for not remembering the night before. I remember sending her the email, but the contents of that email were vague to me. When I read it, I was astounded. I was in the hospital for two weeks while trying to sort out what was going on. I kept telling them I was fine, but my psychiatrist didn't think so. And her word was what kept me there. It sucked.

Midnight Demon

Why I Find Myself Suicidal

When I was in the hospital on a couple of occasions, I was asked why I found myself suicidal. A mental health worker just could not understand why I would want to take my life. So many people think life is precious and taking it is just not right. I won't go into the religious aspect because I lost my faith years ago, and more so when the Catholic Church was harboring pedophiles and did nothing about it for years. But I digress…

Most of the time, I do not know why I want to end my life. I just feel that life is not worth living. I feel so dead inside that continuing to live just does not make sense. Sometimes I feel so dead that I just wish my autonomic nervous system would realize this and stop working, that my heart and lungs would cease to move as they should. But that isn't how it works.

I have not attempted suicide in quite a few years. Maybe it is because when I did, I felt panic that dying was going to happen and it changed me into wanting to live, if only for that moment. But since then, I have changed methods. Now, instead of overdosing on drugs, I plan on putting a rope around my neck or a plastic bag over my head. This is instant death that you can't go back from without some sort of intervention.

Another reason I think about ending my life is because of pain. During my recent hospital stay, I was asked what my pain level was every time I had to take my medication. Yet when I was given my anti-depressant, I was not asked what the level of my depression was. I brought this up to my case worker and she said, "That is what we are talking about…to assess your pain," but she never asked it in a way that I thought was in numerical form. Nor did she ask the level of distress that I was feeling. When given an antidepressant, shouldn't the level of depression be measured? I know that these medications take time to work, sometimes several weeks, but shouldn't a baseline be used to gauge the effectiveness after a week to see if maybe the drug needs to be increased? I was at this hospital for two weeks and never was my psychological pain

Midnight Demon

assessed. My depression and feelings were, but not my psychological pain. It was interesting that my case worker thought there was no distinction of pain versus feelings. I guess in her mind, they are one and the same, but they are not to me.

When you have feelings of killing yourself, the feelings are more than just the typical run-of-the-mill depression that everyone goes through at some point in their life. When you are chronically suicidal, thinking of taking your life every day for months, your feelings have to be so deep and painful that ordinary measures just don't cut it. When you have mental pain, it is like you cannot breathe and have an invisible hundred pound weight on your chest. Taking a deep breath is the only way to get the lungs moving, at least that is how it is with me. Nothing helps this pain and even though I take a narcotic for my physical pain, I do not get relief for the psychological pain. This pain can be defined as the melding of despair, anguish, hopelessness, helplessness, guilt, shame, loneliness, and depression all rolled tightly together in the confines of the mind, which knocks out any kind of joy and pleasure that life might bring. This pain, this ache, is what the father of suicidology, Dr. Edwin Shneidman, called psychache and believed it was the underlying cause of all, if not most, suicides. Stop the psychache, stop the suicide.

This psychache causes the constriction of the mind into believing that there is just one way out of this hell -- suicide. As this pain cannot be relieved by any drug known to man, it is this pain that drives one to think endlessly about suicide. It is this never-ending, all-consuming pain that makes life not worth living. This is what drives the suicidal mind. Ending this pain is what suicide is all about. It is a deep desire to end this suffering of living day in and day out with mind-numbing mental pain. No doctor can treat it. And knowing this makes the hopelessness fuel the pain even more.

Blog Post: What Do You Say?

I have been asked to write about what you say to a person who has just attempted suicide. Well, you try and be supportive and say things like "I'll kill you if you try this again". It is one of the worst things you can say to the person. Being there and hearing the person's story of why they did what they did will be invaluable. It might even prevent another attempt. If this was a one time deal, the person will say that it was the stupidest thing they ever did and may not try again. If they say something about being stupid to think that it was really going to work, and they seem harder on themselves because they survived or are wickedly pissed off, there is a very good chance they will attempt again and again until they succeed. I know this from experience.

I first overdosed when I was sixteen, April 12, 1992. I remember the day as if it was yesterday. I had carefully planned out my pills, the day, how I was going to do it. I even went to confession the day before (I was a practicing Catholic at the time) and went to church on this sunny Sunday. It was my aunt's birthday and I knew that I would have the house all to myself. All I had to do was wait. By the time I got home from church, I knew that my family would be heading over to my grandmother's house, not knowing that I was back home and planning on ending my life. Except it didn't work. I got very sick, puked everywhere, and my eyes were dilated for days.

When I woke up Monday morning, I was pissed off! To my dissatisfaction, I went to school in a very angry mood. I couldn't tell anyone what I had done, nor could I tell them why I was so angry. There was one person I did tell. It was not the school nurse or a friend, but was my therapist at the time…a social worker who, a month or so before, had told me she was leaving the state and I would have to find someone else to take care of my mental health needs.

Midnight Demon

    I don't remember what happened too much the day after, I was still drugged up and out of it, but I remember being so mad at everyone, most of all at myself, because I failed. I then fell into one of the worst depressions of my life. I didn't go to the hospital, as I said I was never going to do it again, so I lied as much as it took to avoid being admitted. The hell with the help. It failed me and I was really, really angry. This therapist was my third and I figured strike three, you're out.

    That summer, I did go into the hospital. I lost twenty pounds, had no appetite, and thoughts of killing myself were rampant. I felt like the biggest asshole on the planet because I failed to kill myself and that kind of pain is hard to describe. You have no idea what failure is until you try and take your life and fail at it. It hurts and that is what I was feeling. This big hurt that no one knew because who would want to know how much it hurt to fail at killing yourself when you thought things out so perfectly. Nobody knew I had done what I did. If they found out, I would be met with concern and would feel more like a burden than I ever did before the attempt. I also felt that nobody would listen to me. I was a pretty good student and who would believe that I was having problems holding things together after my parents had a massive argument that ultimately ended their marriage. I felt that I should have been smart enough to sort through this all by myself.

    I remember on that day, the phone just kept on ringing. I couldn't understand why. Didn't the world know this was my day to end things? I'm not sure if the phone constantly ringing was a good or bad sign. It was my best friend wanting to hang out and I was half in the bag, so to speak, so there was no chance of me leaving the confines of my house to play ball. But I wonder if the panic of what I was doing forced me to throw up all that I had taken. I remember right before falling asleep that this was it. I was going to sleep for the last time.

    There have been at least ten times I have tried to end my life since then. Unfortunately, I don't always remember what was happening with me when I was just about to do it. What I do remember, and it is still the case today, that most of my attempts have been planned and not impulsive. I did have an impulse the first time I truly wanted to die as I took a pair of scissors and tried to dig out a vein and die that way, but that was a lot harder than it seemed. I was introduced to cutting, which can also look like a suicide attempt, especially when the cuts are deep. Though I am a former self-harmer, that is not the subject of this book and I will defer commenting on that for now.

The reason I had first cut was because I wanted to die. I had tremendous stress with a parent that day and I just snapped. All I could think about was death. Up until that time, I was the perfect student in my high school freshman year. I was getting all A's, and nearly had a perfect attendance record. After this blowout, I didn't care too much about anything. My grades slipped and my attendance faltered. I entered therapy and discovered more than I bargained for. I could not let anyone in on the hurt I was feeling. I had grown up with "What goes on in the house, stays in the house".   I just wanted the pain to end so I had cut to end it. Fortunately, I wasn't a good cutter and all I did was cause scratches on my wrist. It wouldn't be until a year later that I would make my first serious suicide attempt.

Like my pain that I tried to hide, I also kept my visible scars hidden. Today they are a reminder of how bad things were and that I survived. I know it may sound strange, but they are truly what saved me from attempting more serious attempts on my life. Planning an attempt was not as easy as it sounds, but it was what has kept me going. It was my escape hatch and, although a lot of researchers have written about suicide as an escape, it truly can be as good as I know it to be. I have thought of many plans, but have not acted on any since before 2001. That makes over a decade of planning, yet no action. You might think that I have been lucky but, in 2005, I came close to acting on my plan.

Things were going pretty crappy for me emotionally and I was still struggling with my nerve injury. Chronic pain and depression do not mix. It

Midnight Demon

seemed that both liked to feed off one another and I was swimming in both physical and mental anguish. I could barely keep above water so I created this wonderful plan, set a date, and all I had to do was get my affairs in order by Nov 5th, 2005. However, the one thing I was counting on, fooling my therapist into thinking I was okay, failed horribly. The way she recounts it today is "Always be aware of someone making an effort at feeling good". This is true. The moment someone in a deep depression suddenly starts to feel better is the crucial time to ask about suicidality. The reason being is that this provides the sufferer relief. The so-called "warning signs" of suicide can be just that...suddenly feeling better after a deep depression and giving away possessions. These warning signs are subtle to the outside observer. Even a trained professional could miss them. I was under siege with suicidal thoughts, yet no one knew until the day my therapist asked what was really, really going on. If not for her insight into my care, I probably would not be here today writing this.

It is important to realize that the attempter does not want people to find out about their plan, especially when they have been thwarted many times in the past with hospitalization after hospitalization. Statistically, I should not be here but, as my therapist points out, I am the exception. Why? I do not know. But holding my thoughts to myself was my haven. I thought carefully about my plan every day and that brought me some relief from my pain.

Constant vigilance is key after someone attempts suicide. If they are intent on ending their lives, they will try and try again until they succeed. If the suicide was a "wake up call", and if they truly get the help they need, they may not try again. But these types of preventions are not always sound. What holds true for one may not hold true for another. The biggest thing to worry about with attempters is the amount of guilt and sense of failure after the attempt that makes another attempt all that more eminent.

As mentioned earlier, hearing the person's story is the most important thing you can do before or after an attempt. Just listening without being judgmental and criticizing can be important for the person, and might be just the thing to prevent another attempt. There is a book called Building a Therapeutic Alliance with a Suicidal Patient by Konrad Michel and David Jobes, two of the foremost suicidologists in the world. They have written an awesome account of how to build an alliance with a suicidal person. It should be the textbook guide to anyone in the mental health field. It gives case studies of clients and the therapist's reaction, good and bad. If you are reading this and are a mental health professional, I strongly urge you to get this book. I have studied the works of David Jobes for several years now. You might even call me a professional stalker as all I do is literature searches on him at least every month to find out what new study he has done with his works on Collaborative Assessment and Managing Suicide (CAMS). In this work, the SSF (Suicide Status Form) is the key element to help a survivor or someone who is about to attempt suicide to help work through their issues on why they think ending their life is the key to solve their problems. But without knowing the story behind the pain, no one will be able to help this person that has just attempted to end their life.

    In my story mentioned above, you can see how much pain I was in that caused me to think ending my life was the answer. While being in this bubble of hopelessness and despair, no good feelings can penetrate it. I guess that is why my therapist crossed the boundaries and told me she cared. When she started crying, I knew that to be true. Hearing the person tell you why they are thinking about ending their life is so essential to *saving* that life. To reassure this person that they are not a burden, not a bother, is the most important thing you can do to try and help bring some hope and ease the pain. There is really nothing more than you can do to help this person, but just knowing you are there and that you are not going to leave or think

Midnight Demon

less of them can help save this person from making another attempt.

I have been through some very close calls. One attempt was medically serious and I was forced into the hospital for three months because a therapist, who was more than pissed off at me, was so very certain I was going to try again. And I would have had I not given myself some time to heal while under the hospital's care. I was in a very dark place and there was no other way out of my abyss. I had tried all the medications, but they didn't help me. I tried therapy for years and it didn't help me. After all this time and energy of trying to plan the end of my life, I still try and hold on to some hope that there will be a better tomorrow. Sometimes there is and sometimes things are the same. This hurts. Knowing day after day that there is no way out other than suicide is a very lonely place, a place that is filled with hurt. I had tried and I failed again. There is no greater pain than that.

I have learned from my mistakes. I have learned not to trust people, especially mental health professionals. I learned that if you tell them of your suicidal plans, they will try and stop you from achieving those ends. I honestly have no idea how my therapist can deal with me sometimes because I am hell bent on ending my life. I think she lives in a fairytale world where suicide doesn't exist because her answer is always an emphatic "no". But could it really be a "yes"? If all therapists were to "green light" their client's suicide, there would be no hope for prevention. But therapy is still supposed to help those in need and yet, after more than fifteen years in therapy with different modalities, I still remain depressed and suicidal. Though I might get a respite every now and then, it is too few and far between to really count. I have learned not to hold on to it because that usually means a big downfall and another hospitalization.

Now I find myself writing about every attempt I have made and the consequences of those actions. I don't know if that is what people want to read, but I write about the aftermath and how it felt after each failed attempt. Maybe I have just given up on trying to attempt again and that is why it has been so long since I have. True, I feel like the biggest failure in the world knowing this. How can I not? It's deeply personal when I talk about the lowest point in my life and wanting to end it all and then, by some grace, still be forced to live on afterwards because of some kind of divine intervention. Of the many attempts, only one was medically serious to warrant a hospitalization. The others were not as serious, but did lead me to be hospitalized. Since the age of sixteen, I have had close to thirty hospitalizations. Most have been involuntary, as I posed a danger to myself and it is state law to hospitalize for that reason. I just wonder why I have survived this long.

Am I still considered suicidal if I don't attempt and just plan? We can go into the whole what makes a person a suicidal ideator versus an attempter, but most would agree that prevention lies before the attempt, not after. We hear stories about suicides and their family's loss, but what you don't hear at all is about the attempter that survived. These truly are the ones that need the most attention, but because their world is so private, no one really knows. Unless someone survives a shotgun wound, immolation (setting oneself on fire), or hanging attempt, you often don't see the scars of attempters. Those that slice their wrists leave scars, but most survive to eventually tell their tale. There are countless overdoses every year that get under-reported or, if successful, get ruled as accidental poisonings rather than suicide mostly to either spare the family the shame, or because there was no clear indication that the poisoning was intentional. Most people believe that unless there is a suicide note, it is not a suicide because he or she wouldn't do that. I would say that the majority of people who attempt and fail feel too ashamed to admit what they have done and cover their asses by saying it was an accident or just a foolish impulse. However, for those that succeed, we will never know.

Talking about an attempt is difficult for the survivor. They really need support after the attempt. I know not all family members are supportive when it comes to mental illness. When someone they love and care about just tried to take their life, fear of losing them overtakes the care and compassion that they might feel. I know that, with my family, I did not have that kind of support. I felt like a burden to most of my family because I had this illness I could not control that was causing me to feel like the scum of the earth.

If you are reading this and truly want to help someone after an attempt…whether it be a friend, co-worker, or family member…do not shy away from them. Let them know how much they mean to you and look them in the eye when you do. This person feels so out of it, they do not want to come back to the land of the living. The shame and the guilt is killing them in ways the attempt never did. If they thought that killing themselves was the answer, they may now know that it is not. If the attempt caused an injury, that will be even harder to deal with. Not only have they failed to kill themselves properly, they injured themselves. That will be hard. Saying they have their whole life in front of them or that they were lucky to survive will only make them feel worse. I still don't feel lucky to have survived my attempts. I still feel ashamed of myself and like the biggest failure in the world.

Blog Post: Voices and Other Musings

I don't know why I am writing this as I am very tired and want to go to sleep, but the voices are having conversations in my head about things. Some stuff I can decipher, others I cannot. It is very annoying. I wish they would just go away and let me be, but they are not so accommodating.

I have lowered my dose of my anti-psychotic because I was having side effects. I don't think I can go back up without my doctor's okay. I just need a little time to adjust to this dose and I am hoping the voices will go away. Something tells me that is just wishful thinking. I really don't want to go back into the hospital. I won't have my music to listen to and having music with me calms me down. I will get agitated if I don't have music and…well, you don't really want to have a meltdown on a psych unit. It is not pleasant. I guess as long as I am not feeling paranoid, I am doing okay. But, I don't have too much interaction with people I don't know.

I am stuck in my house because my funds for Starbucks have ended. I can't have my coffee until next week when my paycheck gets in. It's just as well because I think the caffeine might have had something to do with the tremors I was experiencing. I have been okay the past few days, but I still get the feeling like my arms are, like, stretched out rubber bands. I know that is a little of the dyskinesia I experience. I am also worried that this feeling is going to drive me nuts more than the voices will.

In case you are reading my blog for the first time, I have been hearing voices since the age of five. They started off as imaginary friends, but have stayed with me growing up. The voices have changed over the years. My latest new voices have an English accent. I think that was because I was preoccupied with England for a time. For the most part, they have gone away, but sometimes still creep back.

Midnight Demon

    I also have experienced paranoia while on the bus. I thought it was anxiety, but if anxiety caused paranoia, why would I think one of the passengers was going to harm me in some way? I have not been taking the bus that often anymore because of this.

    Sometimes I have delusions. When I was younger, I had delusions that I was living on the holodeck on the Enterprise. I created this other life that I still somewhat believe today. Or I wish it still existed. Lately, my delusions are related to the type of voice I hear. If the voice says he is Allah, I will have religious-type delusions. Usually, these new voices are often commanding (they tell me to do things) and always lead to a hospitalization. I don't know why voices are an automatic reason for getting hospitalized. I just know that I could be okay otherwise, but as soon as I say I have voices that are not controlled, they put me in the hospital. It drives me nuts…no pun intended.

    Other delusions that I have had in the past centered around my co-workers conspiring to fire me or have me fired by planting devices in my email. I felt like every move I made was being watched and every email I sent was being monitored. Usually, it would center around one person. And, eventually, I became fearful of this person, although I had no real reason to be. When I seriously asked my co-worker if she was going to kill me, she gave me a crazy look. I then knew that it was just my illness talking and that it wasn't real.

    The hard part about dealing with psychosis is that your view of reality becomes blurred. You often don't know what is real and what is not. There was a period of time when I thought God was always watching me and that I had to watch what I was doing so as not to offend him. These feeling persisted and, even when no one was in the room with me, I still felt his presence. It was not a good feeling. I felt like I was constantly being watched, and the voices helped to confirm my suspicions. It wasn't until I started on the drug olanzapine that all this went away. For the first time in my life, I felt free. But then, out of fear of me getting diabetes, my psychiatrist took me off this drug. I was fearful that this paranoia was going to come back, but it has been over ten years and, so far, I am still free from that type of paranoia.

    I often wonder how other people react when someone tells them that God is all around them. For me, I ended up with paranoia for most of my childhood and early adulthood. And it all stopped by taking my medication. I was on other anti-psychotics at this time, but none of them took care of that presence I felt all the time. It feels good knowing you don't have to always watch over your shoulder. That is why I am fearful that I might have to stop this medication. I haven't had any symptoms since Monday and I hope it stays that way. It doesn't make sense. If the symptoms were specific enough, like fine motor tremors, I would have chocked it up to low blood sugar and not be freaked out as much. Since that day, I have not had another episode.

    I see my psychiatrist tomorrow. I hope she has answers for me that don't include me being taken off my medication. So far she has not responded to the emails I sent her so I am hoping that by reducing the dose, I am doing the right thing. But I also hope that doesn't mean it's open season on a voice attack or that paranoia will start coming back. I am just fearful of this happening. But I think if she really wanted me off this medication, she would have responded and told me so.

Midnight Demon

My Therapist

We talked about a couple of issues while she was gone that I had texted her about. I had to keep her in the loop while she was away. I don't know who else's therapist does that.

Friday, I was telling my psychiatrist that I was lucky to have her and not to have her drop me when she was going through all the moves that she was making. I didn't connect with anyone while trying to find another therapist that was closer to me. My psychiatrist did bring up a point that I didn't drop either one (my therapist or my psychiatrist), though I did try to drop my therapist many times. It just never worked out. And today, I see why. She really cares about me, but I think her hounding and nagging isn't helping. We talked about that today after she tried to assess my suicidality. I told her I was fine, but she didn't believe me. She never does. And it pisses me off because sometimes I really am fine.

I have known her for the past 12.5 years (technically 13 if you count the initial session we had). I had an initial session with her in Aug 2000, but because she didn't take my insurance, I had to wait till January to see her. It was a trying time. I was in severe back pain because I had a herniated disc. I was severely depressed because the therapist before her had just left me after a year of working together. I was hurting because I had just broken up with my girlfriend. I was seriously thinking of killing myself because feelings of abandonment were running rampant and I didn't know if I wanted to go back to therapy. I had so many therapists over the course of 10 years, and I wasn't going to go again just to get hurt. But something in her demeanor made me think that she was the one. And now, after all this time, I realize that we have a lifetime commitment to one another (well, maybe not, but it feels like it!).

When I first heard the song by Terri Clark, "First to Fall", it was the perfect song for the beginning of our relationship. I was just getting over my relationship with a previous therapist and I

Midnight Demon

didn't know if I would continue with therapy. I was going out on a limb, trying my luck with Bozo.

I didn't always call her Bozo. I used to call her by her formal title, Dr. E. But, as the years went by, she wanted me to call her by her first name, A. Her middle name starts with a B., but I didn't know it for the longest time. And it is an unusual name. So I just started calling her Bozo hoping that she would get mad at me and stop seeing me. It turned out that no matter what I called her (including some explicit language), it never changed her mind. And wasn't I in trouble!! She and I had a connection from day one. I like to think that it was the song by Kenny Chesney, "You Had Me From Hello" that explains it all.

I don't know how I got to be lucky enough to have this woman in my life and have such a good relationship with her. It took a long time to trust her, especially after dealing with the diagnosis of Cauda Equina Syndrome. That diagnosis brings such a loss of dignity that you cannot imagine what it is like until it reaches you. But through all of my illnesses, she has been there.

I feel like I can talk to her about anything now. I just wish I could talk to her about the grief that I feel at times. It is not an easy thing to admit and it is a painful process.

She doesn't have a traditional track, like CBT or psychodynamic. She has what is called "relational therapy". I am guessing she picked it up back in New Mexico because I can't seem to find out about it anywhere else. She really wants to know me as a person and not just as a diagnosis. I think if she were a strict therapist, I might not be with her after all this time. Even though I might not have frequent sessions, we still are able to "read" each other on the phone by the sound of our voices. I can see the faces she makes when we talk although, for a long time, I rarely had any type of eye contact. I think our phone sessions have increased our eye-to-eye contact more than it has in the past. It helped break the barrier of what I felt I couldn't talk about and really start talking about it. She also allows me to have input in the kind of treatment I want. If I didn't bring in the works of Dr. Shneidman or Dr. Jobes, I doubt that I would be here today. She altered her practice style for me and I never took that for granted. Her style might be considered eccentric, but it works for me. I am grateful that she allowed the use of the SSF and a psychological pain scale for measuring my psychache. I even think that if I brought in the most ridiculous form of therapy, she might just be game because *she* has brought some ridiculous forms of therapy to *me*.

Midnight Demon

Start of Suicidal Career: The Beginning

I don't remember the first time suicide entered my vocabulary. I think it was around the time I was eight and found out my cousin, who was young, killed himself from a drug overdose. I had a lot of cousins in the early eighties that were into drugs. I also had a cousin that shot himself when I was really young, around the age of two. All these cousins were on my mother's side of the family. As far as I know, there is no known mental illness on my father's side…other than, perhaps, depression.

I don't know why suicide fascinated me. I thought it would be cool to be dead. I wouldn't have to go to school anymore or listen to my parents fight over small stuff. By the age of ten, I was calling suicide hotlines. At first, they thought I was joking. How could a ten-year-old want to kill themselves? And how, exactly, would I do it? The operators always got mad when I called, thinking I was calling for attention or a prank. But they didn't know the emptiness that I felt and how much I just wanted to escape. My parents fighting got worse as I got older. It was usually over money. We were poor, on welfare, and could barely keep up with household bills. At least that was what the fights were about. Even though my parents always had food on the table, I remember my father flipping out if my mother spent more than two hundred dollars on monthly groceries. I never understood why. It wasn't like she was buying frivolous things. It was food we needed.

As I grew up, the more I started to loathe myself because I just felt like a burden to my family. I was starting to develop, and I didn't like it one bit. I really felt uncomfortable in my own skin. No one knew this. It wasn't until many years later, after I became an adult, that I really comprehended what was going on. Now I wish I spoke up when I was growing up. Maybe things would have been different for me and I wouldn't have had to cut my wrists or other parts of my body because I was so disgusted with myself. I am talking about gender dysphoria. I still believe that I am a male,

Midnight Demon

although it seems I have made some adjustments so that I don't hate myself as much.

Since kindergarten, I knew that I was different. I didn't realize I liked women, though. That came about when I was in my late teens. I had attractions to women on the subway and I couldn't understand it. I thought I was going crazy and if I brought the subject up with my therapist, I thought I would have been committed to the hospital indefinitely. I was so scared and I didn't have a friend I could talk to about this so I just held it inside. It wasn't until I blacked out while I was cutting myself did I realize just how painful I really was feeling because I liked females. I did a good job on my wrist, cutting myself over thirty times. It wasn't until I was going to cut a vein that I snapped out of it. I looked at what I had done and couldn't believe it. I knew I did it, but I didn't believe that I did it. It felt surreal. I was seventeen at the time. At first, I didn't tell anyone what I did.

It was Martin Luther King's birthday and we had the day off from college. I somehow brought it to the attention of the school nurse and told her I was not "present" when I did this. I was so scared I would go back to that blackout and try to kill myself. My mother was called and I ended up back in the hospital. It was there that I met another patient who was homosexual. He told me it was normal for me to feel this way. It was really a load off my mind. I never felt freer. I came out while I was in the hospital, even telling my treatment team I was gay. And they didn't commit me to life on the unit. They were okay with it. That night, I was so happy that I decided to tell my best male friend...except he wasn't so accepting. He thought I was crazy. He couldn't believe that I liked women. I dissociated to the point of being catatonic. I was hearing voices telling me I was a lowlife and that I should kill myself, but I couldn't speak. I had to go back on my anti-psychotic medication to bring me out of it. It helped with the voices.

Coming out to my friends or family was not so easy. I was so giddy and happy that I could be so free, but I wasn't sure my friends at college would be so accepting. The change in my personality was huge. I was happier than I had been my whole life, at least for a little while. I told my best female friend in school. She was accepting. She didn't care. But I still had trouble with my other friend, Tony. I had known him since we were in diapers. To lose his friendship over this hurt like hell, but we got through it by not bringing the subject up. He thought having sex with me would change my mind, but we had already tried that previously and I could never perform with him. I love him too much like a brother. Besides, it actually turned me off to be intimate with a male partner.

I had a hard time telling my family. My sisters and I had the same circle of friends and if my friends knew, there would be a chance that it got back to one of my sisters. So, one night, I told my sisters that I was gay. I thought my little sister was okay with it, but she really wasn't. My middle sister was more accepting. With my mother, on the other hand, it was tough. To be the first born and be gay was really hard for her to comprehend. I had always admired boys, most likely because I wanted to *be* them, and had a few "crushes" while in middle school. I never hooked up with any boy. It just wasn't my thing. I prefer the company of boys over girls because I feel like one of the guys, but that is as far as it goes. There were a few females in my class that I really liked, but I was shy and insecure and I knew that they liked boys so there was no way for me even to dream about approaching them without getting my ass kicked.

After I came out in high school and to my sisters, I had to tell my mother. It was very difficult. She accepted me, but didn't believe me. It really hurt, especially when she expected me to give her grandchildren. That wasn't going to happen as I had no intention of having kids. Of course, I never thought about getting married or being in a long-term relationship with someone because I always feared my mental illness would kill me. I think it took time for my mother to accept me for being gay. We still don't talk about it, ever. But I think there is a little more acceptance as I have gotten

Midnight Demon

older. When Ellen DeGeneres came out on national TV, we watched it together and not one word was said about it.

I never told my father that I was gay. I think he figured it out before I did, at least that is what a cousin told me a few years ago. My father and I don't have a good relationship. We tolerate each other. I don't call him, but he will sometimes call me, usually when he is having a medical problem of some sort. I keep my distance with him because he gets on my nerves very quickly. I don't trust him. He has abused me for the last time. To most people, he seems like a nice guy. He is a narcissist bastard. He only cares about one thing -- himself. He'd rather buy a $300 dollar suit than pay the utilities. This was what I had to grow up with. This was why I can't stand being around him. And there was no talking to him about it. In his eyes, he is a good father. That is all I am going to say on the matter.

My mother was passive. She allowed anything as long as it was within her norm. I don't get along too well with her because I have a lot of anger for marrying my dad and allowing him to rule the household when he was too immature to do a good job of it.

Daily Living Activities

    I live in a depressed state most of the time. It takes me a long time to get dressed and make decisions about what to wear…from the socks to the pants/shorts to the shirt, etc. But the thing that I always have to psych myself up for is a shower. It should be an easy decision, but because I have to stand longer than I should, it is painful. Instead of being invigorating, it actually exhausts me, both physically and mentally. I rarely love taking a shower. I have such a bad association with it because I just want to crawl back in bed afterwards. It takes too much energy sometimes just to put clothes back on. It takes everything out of me. I don't think that it is a good thing to be exhausted after showering, but I usually am and I have grown to despise it. I don't even stay in long, maybe ten minutes, yet it still robs me of the energy for the day.

    However, if I take it at night, sometimes it wakes me up and then I am up until all hours of the night. It really is mind-boggling how a shower affects me. You know you need to do it because of good hygiene and all, but sometimes I just want to stay away from it because it bothers me so much. I usually try and take a shower every 2-3 days or so. I do this because my mother is always bitching about the water bill so that further causes me to wait until I am raunchy and smelly before I take one. It is better in the winter, but the summer sucks. I sweat and you have to take a shower more just to get the stuff off you. I am lucky my hair is short and I don't go out much because it gets greasy looking. Once it starts itching, I know I have no choice but to shower. I know you might think that this is silly, but it really gives me anxiety.

    I guess my pain medication has kicked in enough for me to try and shower. It will do one of two things…either wake me up, or tire me out.

Midnight Demon

Blog Post: Hodgepodge of Blogs

I am feeling a little lost. I was supposed to kill myself today. That was the plan for the longest time. And, like I thought, I don't feel like killing myself. But that doesn't mean that I am not suicidal. I just feel like I let myself down again. I don't know why I bother saying I am going to kill myself if I am not going to go through with it. I think I just played the "cried wolf" card so many times that I actually don't think I am capable of killing myself, despite coming up with elaborate plans to do so. All that planning has gone to waste. I find it depressing that I am not living, yet I can't die. I really wish my body would wake up and realize how dead I feel all the time. I can't feel happiness. I can't feel joy. All I feel is this emptiness inside. I really feel that if my feelings were connected to my autonomic system, maybe I would have the chance of dying in my sleep.

Ever since I read an article about suicide survivor reaction, I have been thinking about killing myself in the worst way. I am a multi-suicide attempt survivor. I think death is the answer to my problem, yet I am still here. Now, that could be because my reasons to live versus my reasons to die ratio is not high enough, or because I suck at trying to kill myself. Another reason is that I am not meant to die yet, but I digress. There were nights I hated myself for surviving my attempts and I still do. According to all the research, I should be dead. My therapist calls this an exception to the rule. Maybe I am, but I still try to plan my death.

Suicide attempters can be a challenge to clinicians. How do they deal with this population that is at risk for attempting again? Research suggests that asking how they feel about their attempt might be useful.

I was not glad that I survived the attempt. I was not feeling ambivalent. But I think some people do have these thoughts and they go on living. Yes, they have attempted it, but it also brought to them a realization that they were glad they survived. This was something I have never experienced.

Midnight Demon

Reactions to how an attempter feels afterwards can be an important clinical assessment, but something that might not be used across all clinicians. In this assessment, it could perhaps lead to preventions because suicide attempters are more likely to try again. Maybe if we ask how they felt when they first survived, we might find a clue and prevent another attempt.

My therapist and I have tried to work on what to do should "Mr. Hyde" show up while she is on vacation. Mr. Hyde is the side of me that comes out when I'm deeply suicidal and want to write suicidal goodbyes. He may not text or call for help. But, the thing is, other than feeling really suicidal, he doesn't feel the need to ask for help. I feel totally normal when he emerges. I go about my business like I normally do. Except I am writing dark stuff and planning the end of my life. I am beyond hopeless so what would be the point of reaching out? I don't feel the need to talk to anyone. All I need is a pad and pen, or my laptop and I am good. I express all the dark stuff on paper or send off messages to people that I care about telling them I love them and not to worry. That I will be in a better place. It seems normal to me, but I know it's not normal when I wake up from this dissociative state. Only when I am out of it do I really feel the sting of the pain because I am still living. During these episodes, I really feel that I am going to die, that I will fall asleep and not wake up. Then I wake up and wonder if I dreamt all that, but then the yellow legal pad or messages I get in the morning tell me that it wasn't a dream. That I wasn't in my "right" mind, at all.

I think the stigma around suicide needs to change. People need to be able to think about it like they do vanilla ice cream. They either like it or hate it but, regardless, vanilla ice cream is still going to be around. As long as there are conscious people, there is going to be suicide. It might be thought about by people that are in chronic pain and suffering from depression. It might just be that the person is suffering from depression and they just feel like they cannot go on. They might have voices telling them they should not be around or should just disappear. Or maybe the voices just tell them to kill themselves because they will be better off. But I do know this…people should be open to suicide like they are to ice cream. They should hear the person that is bringing up thoughts of death and thoughts of killing or harming themselves. The stigma needs to stop. The hurting needs to stop. I don't know if this blog will make sense and reach the people it needs to. As long as I am here and not in the grave, I hope that people will read this and know they are not alone. The feeling of being able to talk openly about this needs to happen. Too many people feel they are crazy and they don't need to be. Too many people seek help and are denied that help because they have suicidal thoughts. They just need an understanding ear and an open mind.

So the next time someone is thinking about death or talking about killing themselves, I hope that you hear their story as to why they think this is the best way because hearing their story is going to be the deciding factor on whether that person lives or dies.

Sometimes I think that everyone would be better off without me. The only thing that is keeping me alive these days is my word to my therapist that I won't go acting on my thoughts. The pain of living is just too much to bear right now. My therapist often asks me how I get through this. There is a quote that I keep telling her that I got from Hector Berlioz -- "Only one option left…to suffer". I know it doesn't make sense to suffer all the time, but millions of people out there do it everyday. We few that are in this group do it every day, although we come from different backgrounds and sections of the world. I know it sucks, but the trick is to realize that when we feel this way, it is NOT our true selves. It is the disorder that is talking. I know we all feel like scum of the earth for no reason other than for being allowed to breathe.

One reason I have read so much about depression, and there are a lot of good books out there, is that you have to know and understand the disorder, then you can know what to do. Sometimes

Midnight Demon

knowing the demons is better than not knowing them. I know that it isn't always easy when our physical bodies wreck our lives and we no longer feel a part of the human race because our bowel and bladder are not functioning and we have physical pain that is driving us insane. But things aren't always going to be this way. One of the books that I had read said that suicide is usually complete in ten minutes and if you wait out those ten minutes, you will survive. The same thing goes for depression. Though, instead of ten minutes, it's more like ten days. But it doesn't last. Eventually it lifts, and we return to "normal" functioning until the next episode. The hardest part of this disorder is that we forget that we have survived the worst of it. Every time we are stuck in an episode, we think that we are never going to feel better. I am telling you that you are. No matter how hopeless you feel right now, tomorrow might be a better day. If it is not, at least you survived today. Worry about tomorrow. Tomorrow I'll be here for you. Count on it.

Whenever I Have This Pain, I Freak Out

It is easier for me to write about how suicidal I am than to talk about what is causing me to be suicidal. Most of the time, I don't know why I want to kill myself. I just do. I want to escape from the pain, either the physical or the mental. Lately, it has been the physical pain I want to escape from. It's hard to do anything when your foot hurts and you can't do simple stuff like walking. But the last few months, it has not been as bad as it was a year ago. No one knows why I have the pain. They call it tendonitis, but if it were as simple as that, I would have recovered by now. I have seen many doctors over the past two years. I keep seeing my primary care doctor to get my pain medication. If I didn't have my pain medication, I would not be here writing this book. Chronic pain changes you. It takes so much out of you mentally and physically.

I often miss things because I can't stand too long or walk too far. If I overdo it, I can be incapacitated for up to three days, depending on the severity of the pain. In early April of this year, I went to my little cousin's wedding. She is an adult, but she is younger than I am so I call her "little". She is my second cousin on my father's side. The day she got married, I wasn't feeling too confident that I could attend, but I pushed through like I always do. I stood for what seemed like hours and even danced a couple of dances.

It took me three days to recover from that night. I spent the first day in bed and I thought I was fine, even though my ankle bone was the size of a golf ball and my toes were little Vienna sausages. Monday came and I decided to go out. I got half-way down the block when back to bed I went to ice and elevate my foot/ankle. My little excursion cost me another two days. When I came back to the house, I could barely make it up the stairs to my room. I was so incapacitated with pain. It was so bad that I thought about ending my life.

At this time, I was planning on ending my life anyway. I had made a vow to myself that I would not

Midnight Demon

make it until my next birthday. I had enough of dealing with being in so much pain that I could not walk, stand, or go up the stairs. I am fairly young and there is no reason why I am hurting so much. Well, there is a reason: nerve damage. It is the only reason I can think of that could be causing me such agony. What doctors don't get is that this is what my life has become. My days of walking a mile are over. I don't know if I will ever be able to walk long distances again. And because walking is my main mode of transportation, I rely on my feet. To get to faraway places, I use public transportation. It is sometimes a pain because I have to take a bus to take me to where I need to go. I find it disheartening. I used to be able to walk anywhere I needed to go and now I am lucky to walk four blocks at a time. The pain is erratic. There is no rhyme or reason for it to flare up. Sometimes it is because I do too much. I have tried to figure out what I can and cannot do, but the "rules" keep changing. What I am able to do today, I cannot do tomorrow. I have to have rest days in between and I know I am tired because I usually sleep most of the day.

Going to doctor appointments where I used to work is tough. Getting there always exhausts me. I would love to just hang out in the lab and see my former co-workers, but it takes too much energy to go. It also is very emotional because I still have not come to terms with not being able to work.

Every time I think I can rejoin the work force, I have a setback. Some nights I don't fall sleep until morning. I get so wound up that I will be up all night. Sometimes it is due to pain; other times, it is because of anxiety because of my pain. When all this started, I had left foot/leg pain. It was the beginning of my CES. So whenever I have this pain, I freak out. My post-traumatic stress disorder takes over and I can't sleep, even if I take a little Ativan. My brain just refuses to shut down. I am in hypervigilance mode, watching to make sure it doesn't get worse. It takes a lot for me to calm down. I usually end up writing about it in my blog or I write a letter to my therapist. Mostly, if I get into a dark place, "Mr. Hyde" comes out and I usually end up writing dark, goodbye letters. I usually have no recollection of having done it until the next morning when I find the legal pad.

One of my favorite letters written by Edgar Allan Poe describes the struggle of darkness so eloquently. I was talking with my therapist about this and she thinks I dissociated into "Mr. Hyde". I'm still trying to remember what triggered me. I had been depressed most of that day. My first blog was me writing about how I was tired of living. I don't know if that is what set me off or if it was my never-ending menstrual cycle. Though I don't think you can call it a cycle at the present time because it has gone on for weeks now.

The depression, a word I forgot that describes me, has stifled my existence and is trying to extinguish me. These blackout dissociations are one clue that I am not with it. But the problem becomes how to deal with it. Hospital will only treat the symptoms of my depression, and there are no medications for dissociation. I still think that it is just a symptom of my suicidality. I am far too depressed and have crossed over into the blackness of existence. I may not feel suicidal all the time but, on an unconscious level, I still am. Or maybe it is subconscious. Either way, I don't know what to do about it. I am sort of scared that I might try to end my life while in this state. It most likely will be an impulsive move. And, with that, I won't have my crisis response plan to use. I will only be focused on whatever it is I am feeling at that moment and how to get rid of it. Luckily, the midnight demons have only been writing about the end of my life. I don't think I have attempted anything because I'm still here and there are no empty bottles of pills, knife or razor wounds, or ligature marks to indicate to me that I have tried something.

The mind is very complex. It can focus on writing something very emotional, yet can still listen to music as you write. I really want to try and see if the Neurontin (a medication that deals with neuropathic pain) that I take has been the cause of the dissociations that I have been experiencing. But I am afraid that if I do experiment and stop taking it and something were to

Midnight Demon

happen, I won't remember it. I barely remember that I took the pills to begin with so, obviously, something was brewing before I took my dose. I don't take the Neurontin on a daily basis. I usually just take it when the burning sensation is too much or if I want to zone out. But lately, the zoned out part has not worked for me the last couple of times I have taken it.

So now you know how the midnight demons came to be named, although I still don't know what is causing them. I think exhaustion has something to do with it. I am really tired and, instead of sleeping, I just go off into "Mr. Hyde's" world until I do finally succumb to sleep. It just sucks that I am writing very dark stuff before I do fall asleep. I have been lucky so far that I have not done anything. I hope it continues to stay that way. If I am going to kill myself, I want to be in the present state of mind and not be out of it. Or maybe it is better that I am out of it.

Suicide has been an interest of mine since I was young. Now, at nearly thirty years later and I don't know how many attempts, I still think it is the only way out of my suffering. I have made a date this year that, if things aren't improved, I will go through with it. I can't help but think that being dead is the answer to my problems. I know that people say that suicide is the permanent solution to a temporary problem, but my leg pain and depression are not temporary. I have to live with this the rest of my life and if I choose not to, isn't it my choice? Don't I have the right to die if I so choose? I am not saying that I will commit suicide tomorrow, but it is in the future that I will die. I am not promised tomorrow. No one is. I just think that I don't have a purpose. And a lifetime of being in chronic physical pain is not appealing to me. I just can't go on knowing that every day I will be in some kind of pain. Or the fact that I have to be on pain medication for the rest of my life. I just can't fathom that. I worry that, one day, I will be denied the medication because I have been on them for so long. Or that the government will dictate to my doctor what to prescribe. I just can't risk that happening. I'm also afraid of people not believing that I am depressed because I joke around so much. I'm sorry that I have a sense of humor. It has helped me with my depression more than anything. I told my psychiatrist that if I didn't have it, she had permission to commit me somewhere. My heart is so dark at times that I can't stand it. I feel like it should stop beating because I feel so dead inside. And this goes on day after day. There is no relief. I never feel alive and joyful, just sad and despairing.

    I read a lot about Kay Redfield Jamison because I am a huge fan of hers. I like to think that she writes about her life and her experiences as a way to know the beast better. With me, I like to read a lot about suicide and suicide research because I am hoping that at least one researcher will find a way to make me feel better. I think that I am on the right path when I have the works of Edwin Shneidman and David Jobes at my fingertips. I don't think that I would still be here if I hadn't taken that psychometric class in college and searched for an assessment that measures psychological pain. I had researched over thirty articles on suicide risk assessment and none of them came close to Dr. Shneidman's pain scale or Jobes's CAMS model and SSF. I felt like having these instruments were key to knowing myself better and to conquer the demon called suicide.

    I later learned that there is another model similar to CAMS called Aeschi, which I am very fond of. It is under the principle of human connection and knowing the story of why someone is thinking of taking their life that is so instrumental. It might not work all of the time, but it does most of the time. All it takes is an empathic ear.

    And how can we forget William Styron's <u>Darkness Visible</u>. He writes about how depression is like living in a cauldron.

    How many times have we thought that we were wretched and didn't know why? And when we try to explain these feelings to someone, that someone thinks that we must be joking because no one can be in that much agony and still be around to talk about

Midnight Demon

it. Then we have the depression of spirits that, if it should continue, will not fail to ruin you. We all want the despair to end quickly, but it does not. It lingers and hurts and agonizes you until you feel you cannot breathe anymore. We want someone to listen and to help us, and quickly. Not tomorrow, not next week, but today. Now. To lessen the feelings of agonizing despair is something I wish for every day.

Battles With Self

    I talked with my therapist today about a few things. She hasn't gotten the packet of letters that I mailed to her last week so I didn't bring up the subject of grief.

    What I did bring up, I have been wrestling with all day…my transgender issue. I have been born a female, yet my head thinks I am a male. I asked my therapist what she calls me and she said a heterosexual male. My fear is that talking about this is going to stir up some feelings of suicidality. It almost always does because I was not born a male. I just feel that I am one. Coming to terms with this has not been easy. It has only been for the last few years that I have been open about this. I wish I could go back and say when I first started feeling this way and it would be around the time that I was in kindergarten. I started feeling different than other girls. I always liked taking things apart to see how they worked. I didn't like dolls growing up, although I did like trucks and other boy toys. I would love playing over at my friend Tony's house. He had all the cool boy toys. We would play for hours. I was also into a lot of sports growing up, especially baseball. When Tony started to play little league baseball, he was on the Oakland A's. He then decided he was not a Sox fan because he was on the A's. I got mad at him for that because I always felt like you had to root for the home team no matter what.

    During the registration period for little league baseball, I asked my father if I could play. It would have made me the happiest in the world. But my father said no because that was a boy sport. I was so hurt. But I didn't let anyone know how hurt I was. We were poor so I never got the equipment needed, except when a neighbor across the street cleaned out his place and threw away his gloves. It was the first time I actually had baseball equipment. Tony and I played baseball together after college for I don't know how long. When he was off with his team, I would throw the ball against the

Midnight Demon

steps, making diving plays and acting like I was throwing out the runner at second. I played like that for hours. It was really fun. I could hit better than Tony did…I guess because I had a lot more anger than he did. I could also throw the ball farther. We would have contests as to who could throw the farthest. I always won. I also threw the highest. Red Sox baseball became my passion. I would love to watch them play. I didn't go to many games as a kid. Again it was because sports were a boy thing, not a girl thing.

The only sport that I did get involved in was basketball. I might have been able to beat Tony, but I never was good enough to make Varsity. My career high was four points in one game, and that was because only five players showed up. It was a good game as we crushed Brighton. It must have been the first game that I played the whole game, minus the time I spent nursing a calf cramp.

My father and mother never went to any of my games, even though we only lived a block from the high school. They just were not interested. My coach told me I was the shortest player to jump high. That was because there was a high beam between my parent's bedroom and the parlor. I used to always run and jump to see if I could hit it. It took me a long time, but I was finally able to do it, though the downstairs tenants didn't like it much.

Growing up, I looked at all the things that I hated about myself. I hated getting my periods because it caused me so much pain, mentally and physically. I hated developing breasts because I was always bumping into things with them. And it hurt! I never liked the way I looked because of these things. I still don't. I still think I am the ugliest person on the planet. And who could blame me? My father helped by calling me Faccia Brutta ("ugly face" in Italian) every day for as long as I can remember.

I still am not happy with my breasts. I am getting creative and calling them gynecomastia (male breasts) and hoping that if I lose weight, they will shrink. But losing weight is hard when all you want to do is kill yourself.

For a long time, I never put the two together…the being a male and my suicidality. I really had no clue why I was suicidal until, one night, I had the revelation that it could be because I think I am a male and I am not. It is very hurtful to be called a "she" when you want to be called a "he". There was a time that I would always get complemented as a "he" and when the person recognized my gender, they would get all frazzled and apologize. I always said it was okay and that I liked being called a "him". It just felt more natural to me than being called a "her". I can't stand it. And I guess, subconsciously, it was hurting me. It took me to a dark place where suicide became my life's goal. It was all I thought about. Killing myself was the ONLY way out of my situation. If I couldn't be a male and be called "him", then what was the purpose of me living?

    Last year, I decided that I was going to change my name to "Mike". I didn't realize how hard it was going to be. It still is. I told my middle sister this and she was supportive, but scared for me. Flashbacks of when I came out gay as a teenager came flooding back. I couldn't tell my other sister or my mother I wanted to be a male. There would be no way for them to accept me for me. My eight-year-old still asks if I am a guy or a girl and I always answer with, "What do you think"? And then she says I'm a girl. It hurts. I will never forget the day when she came in to the bathroom when I was going and found out the truth. I was crushed. Really crushed. If there was a noose waiting for me that day, it would have had my neck in it. I so wanted to die and still do because I know I can't live my life as a male. I don't really know what that means because, technically, I do live as a male. I wear men's boxers and clothes. The only thing female that I own are underwear and that is when I get my stupid period. I can't go on if I am bleeding monthly. I know this because it kills me to have a monthly. It hurts. And there is no other way to describe it. I can't tell you *why* it hurts. It just does. I have been living this way for most of my life and it kills me when people use the wrong pronoun. I know

Midnight Demon

being open about this will confuse people. I feel like I am causing them a burden and, believe me, I would rather die than cause that grief.

I had a talk with my mother years ago about why I need to buy male things, but it went by the wayside. Even my youngest sister tried to get me to buy women's clothes. I never have liked women's clothes. They just don't fit right. They don't feel right. I wear men's clothes because they are comfortable. My middle sister wanted a football jersey for Christmas last year. She got a men's large, but she didn't like it because it didn't feel right. She wanted me to get her a women's version, but the only jerseys that I could get were men's. Oh, well. I ended up returning it for a medium. Now the football player is in jail for murder so she won't be wearing the jersey anyway!

I wish I could say that I am a female, but it goes against the grain. Even typing the words has my gut twisting in agony. I am a male trapped in a female's body. I do not like it. I hate myself because of it. And I want to take my life because of the shame it has caused me.

The new year started and I thought I could finally come out of the closet and tell my family I'm a guy. Then my menses started and I was really on edge. I told one of my sisters the week after New Years and had a meltdown the whole weekend. I was crying from relief, frustration, anger, you name it. She was concerned about telling my mother and my other sister so I decided to put that off.

Unfortunately, this year has not started right. The week before, the dreaded menses started and have not stopped for the past six fucking weeks. I missed a pill because I was sick and that is how this whole thing started. I am so mad at myself because that is the one pill I take religiously. I have had break-through bleeding and I just want it to stop so I can go back to being a man and wear my boxers. I have to wear female underwear and I don't like it at all. It is messing with my head. Here I was ready to come out as a guy and I am bleeding like a girl. I feel humiliated beyond belief and I want to cut so badly. I'm fantasizing about how it will make me feel, but I know that if I start, I won't be able to stop. It's like a drug. The release is intense. Right now, I'm feeling so numb that it might just help me feel something.

I hate not being able to control my menstrual cycle. I have to go back to the reproductive endocrine doctor. I feel so demoralized, so humiliated because if I was a true man, this wouldn't be happening. I'm so tired of not being a guy on the outside. I'm just about ready to end it all. I have time to write letters to say I am sorry, but my damn cycle fucked everything up for me, and I have to end it. I tried telling my psychiatrist this, but I don't think I got through.

My therapist has my suicide notes I wrote back in 2009. I just gave them to her to hold for me. They were written right before I was involuntarily hospitalized.

I figure if I cut, it might let go some of the suicidal thoughts. I know that sounds stupid, but I really think it might help. I can't stand the pain of living this two lives bullshit anymore. I feel I have taken two steps back in this arena when I wanted to move forward. I hear the constant voice that says I will always be a little girl no matter what, and I want it to shut up once and for all. I won't be graphic about what I will do, but I just think a little cut is all I need to get the stuff out of my head. Maybe then the pain will stop and I can feel normal again.

Midnight Demon

About Hospitals

I thought I would talk about my hospitalizations. In the beginning, I found that most of my hospitalizations were helpful. They helped reset my thinking and took me away from the stress for a little while. It didn't take away all my stress, just enough so I could cope with the demands of everyday life. People think that it is easy to do everything that makes life go round. But when you suffer from depression, you find that even getting up is difficult.

Trying to find something to wear is exhausting. Even taking a shower is sometimes not as exhilarating in the morning as it should be. There were many times after taking a shower that I felt done for the day and I hadn't even started yet. I was always tired. I would have trouble picking what jeans and socks to wear. I had a few pairs of the same shoes so that wasn't a problem. I just grabbed whichever pair was closest to me. I sometimes wore the same pair of jeans for days because I couldn't bear the thought of taking everything out of my pockets and putting it all into the new pair. I did laundry once a month, if that. I just couldn't be bothered. And if I wasn't hungry, I didn't eat. If my alarm didn't go off, I would sleep all day. I got in the habit of taking a shower every other day. Sometimes it would be longer than that. Now that I am no longer working, I can go more than a few days without a shower. Mostly that is because of my pain.

But when you are a patient, all these things are easier. You shower when you want to or are required to. You have a set schedule for eating. You have groups and a routine to follow. It always amazes me that going in sometimes helps me to get back on track and set goals for the day.

But being in the hospital also has its disadvantages. You sometimes have privileges you need to get before you can be discharged. Loss of privileges means more time in the hospital. During the stay after cutting my wrist, I lost a lot of privileges. I didn't cut while in-house, but I thought about it and that was enough to keep me for a few more days. You also didn't have cell phone privileges on some units. That wasn't such a big deal when no one really called me. But I hated it when I wanted to get in touch with my therapist and I had to wait by the floor phone for her to call because if I missed it, it meant I wouldn't talk to her.

There was no communication between the inpatient floor and my outside treatment team. When I was involuntarily hospitalized by my psychiatrist, the inpatient team discharged me without consulting my psychiatrist. I was promptly re-admitted the day that I saw her. She was not in a good mood when I saw her. But I needed to be inpatient because my suicidality was severe. I was at one of the lowest points in my life and was doing things subconsciously. It was around this time that I started talking more about my gender identity. I wanted someone to talk to one-on-one, but they don't do that anymore. You just get this team approach, which sucks. You meet with the attending psychiatrist, social worker, head nurse, occupational therapist, resident psychiatrist/psychologists, and a member of the nursing staff all at once. And, usually, it only lasts for, at most, twenty minutes!! I don't know what they can possibly learn in that twenty minutes. They go a lot by nursing staff reports, which I think are important, but it doesn't help. Sometimes you don't get a check-in like you are supposed to. Some units are strict on setting time aside and meeting with you. At least that's what happened when I was at another hospital unit specializing in trauma.

I was mostly hospitalized because I had thoughts of suicide and was thinking of acting on it. Of the thirty or so hospitalizations that I have had since I was sixteen, four were involuntary, three were because of self-injury (cutting or taking large amounts of medication). When I was eighteen, I had over six hospitalizations during the summer. It was like every two weeks post-discharge, I was back in the hospital. My life was really out of control and lead to me having my first medically serious suicide attempt. I hadn't been that out of control since I was sixteen and was hospitalized every three months.

My depression was one of the lowest it had ever been. I really don't know how I survived. Thoughts of death were constantly with me. I truly felt like I was the lowest human being on the planet. I didn't have energy to look for a job, go to college, or do much of anything. I slept twenty hours a day. When I wasn't home, I was sleeping on the train. Thoughts of jumping on the tracks were rampant. I told my therapist at the time, Dr. B, and she would always hospitalize me. It was the code. Thoughts of suicide always lead to an admission. And I had plenty of thoughts!!

It wasn't until I was in my twenties that I started having less admissions. I realized that I needed them to help stabilize me because my disorder kept me from having a routine I could follow. The hospital recharged my batteries. It took away the every day stress of living, at least for a little while. Some hospitalizations were brief. My shortest one was twenty-four hours. My worst one was at a local hospital that was understaffed and had too many patients that needed one-on-one. One-on-one is when someone needs constant staff assistance because of fear of that individual harming themselves. It was scary and they wouldn't let me have my pens! I freaked out. It wasn't until they called in the on-call psychiatrist that they let me have my pen. I was discharged the next day. I wasn't helped by that hospitalization at all.

I wish I could say hospitalizations have been useful for me over the course of time. They have just been a stepping stone, in my opinion. You stay for a few days or two weeks, usually not longer than that. The only hospital stay that I had more than three weeks was when I overdosed, and it was medically serious enough to warrant a stay longer than two weeks. I was profoundly suicidal. I had nothing to really keep me here and I wanted to die, and the staff knew I had a lethal stash of pills with which to do it. It was a long stay that didn't cure me of anything, but kept me alive to go on to college and set goals for myself.

Midnight Demon

I was still going into the hospital at least twice a year. I called it "maintenance" because I didn't want my suicidality to get too far ahead of me. I was scared to die, but didn't want to live. I still don't. Each day is a struggle with me. Every morning I wake up wondering if today is the day that I am going to fulfill the demons' wishes to die. As the Klingons say, "Today is a good day to die". I never put much effort into it after my failed attempt, though.

A failed attempt is an awful feeling. Since that time, I have learned a trick or two to manage my suicidality. With the help of a couple of pain scales and a suicide status form, I learned to cope better with my pain. But one thing I learned, in October of 2012, is that no matter how much you have a crisis response in place, when you truly want to end your life, you are alone with your thoughts and your feelings and you don't reach out for help.

I survived another mini-suicide attempt because I was in so much physical pain, I couldn't get up to get my bottle of pills to finish myself off. I could not walk the three feet or so to my bureau. It was not scary for me. I wanted my pain to end but, for some reason, I could not get it done because of my immobility. Afterwards, I was kind of in awe that things didn't work out the way I planned. I shocked my therapist and my psychiatrist when I told them. I didn't end up in the hospital, but could have. My psychiatrist knew that it was the pain talking. Another demon to contend with was the chronic pain I have from nerve damage caused by my CES. My therapist wondered why I didn't use my crisis response plan. Frankly, I just couldn't. My mind didn't go there. I didn't assess myself the way I usually do. I had to get rid of the pain and I had to do it now. I hated withering in such agony. It was a terrible feeling. I just didn't know if the pain was going to stop. Pain relievers weren't helping me, at all. In fact, I took a lot of pain relievers that night to try to stop the pain. Eventually, I passed out, out of exhaustion and medication, but it took a long while for this to happen.

I am always fearful of pain flare-ups now. It activates my post-traumatic stress disorder. I start thinking about when I first got CES and all it did to me. I start thinking that this is the end of me because my pain is so great. I wonder when it will end and if my pain medication is going to be enough to hold it at bay. And the worse part is the not sleeping. The longer I am up, the greater my anxiety gets and the more I can't sleep, despite taking Ativan after Ativan. Eventually, the drug does its job and knocks me out, but not until 5 or 6 in the morning.

I was fearful this would be my pitfall, my last stand. That, at last, I met my match and it was all going to be over. In December of 2012, I made a vow to end things if things didn't improve. I did have the ambiguous diagnosis of complex regional pain syndrome so if my pain was not going to be helped anymore, and my depression was not going to get any better, I would end my life before my next birthday. I still have the date in my head and it was just random.

But then I realized that I couldn't do it. My world started falling apart again. The pain increased to the point where I said "Screw December", and my plans for becoming a male were put on hold because I knew my family couldn't take it. I was hurting emotionally and physically. I got involved in a blog site for suicide attempters and found that I was not alone. I wrote for this blog. I started writing this book. And parts of me hoped that I would see it published one day. But I still had a driving need to kill myself. So I pushed the date up.

But then my finances were cut in March of 2013. I no longer had the resources to get away to kill myself because I didn't want my family to find my body. I wanted to die in a hotel room or a secluded place. My plans were all changed and it killed me inside. When I told Bozo my new date, she got all emotional and told me I couldn't kill myself in August or September because those months mean to much to her. She didn't want them tainted with my death. I hated her. I hated everyone that wanted me living.

Midnight Demon

Sadly, I have come to realize that I have to put the needs of others before my own. I am not saying that suicide is a selfish act because it isn't. I am saying that there are people that will be devastated should I kill myself, and I don't want to cause anyone pain, even if I think it will only be for a short while. People are resilient and will get on with their lives. I am the one that has to suffer and live through hell, and I am tired of it. But I made a choice not to continue to live after reading a suicide attempt survivor blog. I know that I will never be content, that my life is always going to be filled with misery.

Blog post: Chronic Pain and Living

I have tried to take my life several times over the years. Currently, I am struggling with the difficulties of trying to stay alive. I keep coming up with plans to end my life. I give myself a date and when that day comes, I plan on ending it. This has been going on for a few years now. My therapist has been able to stop the constriction by telling me how my family will feel and how she will feel if I go ahead and take my life. I can't help making these plans.

I have been depressed for as long as I can remember. I recently have been trying to get at the "root" of my suicidality, but the feelings evade me. I just know that between the ages of 5 and 8, something happened that made me want to take my life. And by age ten, I tried by putting a pillowcase over my head. No one knew about this. I told my mother beforehand that I was going to kill myself, but she did nothing. My confidence in her dwindled that day. I felt I could no longer trust her.

Five years later, I was a freshman in high school and my parents had started World War III. They broke up…and so did my wrist. I started cutting to relieve the psychological pressure and pain. It became my friend over the next seven years or so. At sixteen, I was hospitalized and everyone found out about the voices. That was tough. I had wanted to join the military to get away from my family, but having a psychotic diagnosis, I knew that I never would pass their tests. My career was over before it even started and I fell into a worse depression. I kept on getting re-hospitalized, every three months or so, because I just couldn't handle my life. I was getting worse and the suicidality was getting better. I kept on thinking that I was at the end.

Two years ago, as I was suffering from delusions and psychosis, I had a funny thing happen. I had the voice of Allah tell me that I should sacrifice myself so that the war in Afghanistan

Midnight Demon

would stop. As you probably can tell, I was off my medication again. My psychiatrist didn't think I should be on them all the time because of the side effects. I had to re-start taking them because I was the sacrificial lamb and I believed them. Allah was talking to me and I was the cause of the war of Afghanistan. The only way to stop the war was to stop my life. So I planned another scheme to end my life. Only this time, like before, my therapist stopped me. I tried very hard to get her to see that it had to be done and to think of all the soldiers I would save by ending my life. It seemed like a win. Sacrifice one life so all others could be saved. Isn't that what the military does? Allah was not too happy when I started on my medication again. He was very angry. He also wanted me to end my life because it was better than taking medication. I agreed with him on that, but I couldn't end my life. By this time, I was back in the hospital. I was still delusional, thinking I was the "one" to save it all. But as the medication started working, the delusions slowed down and I began to see more clearly. The voices went away, except for my regular voices that I hear all the time.

Since that time, a lot has changed for me. I have become disabled and am in chronic physical pain. I have a plan to kill myself and it is to happen sometime this year. I have had enough. No pill can adequately control my pain and it is a tough position to live in. I have a condition known as Complex Regional Pain Syndrome (CRPS). It is a neurological disorder in which the nerves are out of whack. No one really knows the cause. I was "lucky" in that I had nerve damage to my ankle already so when I sprained it, twice, I think it allowed that damage to spread. Of course I also don't walk correctly so that didn't help.

I can sit here and give a lecture about pain and suicide, but I am afraid it will fall on deaf ears or not really reach the people it needs to reach. I wish I could say that you can live your life with chronic pain, but I would be lying. There was a time when I was able to. I had adequate pain control and could work a full-time job. That ended when, instead of being placed on a regular psych unit, I was placed in a detox unit and my pain medication was stopped. Since that time in 2002, I have not had adequate pain control and I am afraid to ask for it. I have my pain medication, but it only treats the physical pain. It doesn't help with the burning sensation or the other electrical type pain that I experience. Nothing helps those. No cream or pain gel works. It might be enough to take the edge off so I can sleep, but I am always a 3-4 on a pain scale of 1-10 every single day and when my activity goes up…showering, getting dressed, walking to the bus stop, or standing while waiting for the bus…then the pain also goes up. Sometimes all it takes is my moving my big toe and I am in pain. And with each episode, I think about death. I plan it, I imagine it, I dream of it. I no longer am able to work because I can't walk more than 300 feet. I can't lift things greater than ten pounds. I can't stand more than twenty minutes. And I am only thirty-seven. It is a long battle with CES, and I wish that I could say that not working is helping me. In some ways, it is. It helps me to write and de-stress. My voices are at a lower key than they were when I had a job. I don't have the delusions as much. I just am constantly suicidal. And maybe, one day, I will die by it. But as someone once said, "I am not living and I can't die".

    I have a serious mental illness that wants me to claim my life. I hear voices that taunt everything I do, but I have never been violent towards another person and, god help me, hope I never will. I just want to kill myself because I am a sorry excuse for a human being. I don't blame my parents or my siblings for the way I turned out. It just happens to be who I am. I may not accept it, but it is who I am. I know that, someday, I will ultimately end my life by my own hand. I know because I think about it every day. But I will NOT take another person's life.

    Do I need to have a lifetime commitment because I am so suicidal? Probably, but insurance companies don't see it that way. As long as you are not in "imminent" danger to harm yourself or others, you cannot be allowed to stay in the hospital against your will for more than a few days' time. I have been there many times and even though I have chronic suicidality, I have never been kept beyond the three days - two weeks because of my suicidality. I might have been kept because the voices were telling me to harm myself, but never because I said I was suicidal. The mental health system is wrong and should address these issues. Maybe a longer admission is what I need to get better.

    I have intense psychotherapy with my therapist twice, sometimes three times a week and still feel suicidal. I have been on every drug used for psychopharmacology, yet I still feel suicidal. How am I to live my life when I want to end it so much? How am I supposed to work and go to college when thinking about my death is all that matters to me? No hospital, psychiatrist, or psychotherapist can change it. So the blame gets shifted onto me. It's my fault for not "wanting" to get better; that my negative attitude/emotions are what is causing me to be suicidal; if I change my attitude, I will be happier. It's all bullshit. Being this way is not my fault any more than it's a person's fault because they are dying of cancer. And believe me, I would much rather trade places with them because I know they are going to die, while this "emotional cancer" is eating me alive and no one can see it. And no one wants to help me, either. I can only save myself if I want to.

    Well, I give up. I don't want to live anymore. What purpose will living my life serve? I know it is only going to end up six feet under. I have thought about cremation, but the cost is the same. I thought about buying my own plot somewhere, but I really don't care what my family does with my remains. They are of no use to me anymore. So I am giving myself some time before I do it. And hopefully within this time frame, things will change. Because if they don't, I am dead and there is nothing anyone can do to stop me.

Blog Post: Old Research Journals

    I was going through some old research journals and came across an article on pain and suicide. This was the "first" study to find that moderate to severe pain caused suicide to happen. CLAP, CLAP, CLAP!!! Tell me something I DON'T KNOW. I don't get how they have to do a study in order for doctors and other mental health professionals to realize that any type of prolonged pain (physical or mental) is going to result in suicide. It astounds me, it really does. And the worst part is that these people are not being treated. That's the other thing that drives suicide…untreated pain. Granted, you can't treat psychological pain like you can physical pain. There just isn't a pill you can take to relieve psychological suffering. That is the sad part. But you can assess it. You can hear the person talk about their pain. That is all the person really wants…to be heard.

    Physical pain is ambiguous. And the study didn't focus on any particular pain in the body. The researchers just asked, "Have you had pain in the last four weeks?" and then the subjects rated it. So there is no telling if this pain was coming from the head, back, legs, stomach, etc. Does it matter? I don't think so. I just think that more doctors should ask their patients if they are experiencing pain and how severe it is. And also ask if they are thinking about suicide because of this pain. But most doctors don't have the time to ask these questions.

    For three months after my psychiatric hospitalization, my doctor asked if I was suicidal because of my pain. Then the questions stopped. He began to ask more about what was causing my pain and tried to help me there. A few months ago, he asked me again if I had suicidal thoughts. He then told me that he cared a lot about me and that he would miss me should I kill myself. That caught me off-guard. I know I have a good relationship with my doctor, but do other patients have good relationships with theirs? And are the people that are prescribing

Midnight Demon

narcotics regularly checking to see if their patient is at risk for suicide? My doctor has stopped asking me if the pain medication is adequate for me. Sometimes it is, other times it is not. And I think that finding an adequate pain relief regimen is key to saving a life.

I know that I am constantly complaining on my blog about my pain, but I have pain medication to control it. Even if, at times, it is inadequate. Do I think about suicide? Yes, I do. But I have protective factors that are preventing me from going through with my plan. And I hate these factors because I wish I could kill myself. I know that I will be missed by my blog readers, my family, my therapist, and my psychiatrist. I have a sense of belonging to these people and as much as they drive me crazy, they keep me here. So all I can do is write about my pain and hope that it helps someone to know they are not alone in their pain, too.

The Consultant

Throughout my therapy with Bozo, there have been highs, lows, and plateaus. Sometimes I felt like we were getting somewhere. Other times, I felt we were talking just to shoot the shit. Months would go by and I would feel more and more distant with each session. Then the arguing started a couple of times. Then it was, at least, once a week. We were getting to the point where neither one of us were on the same page. I was getting more and more frustrated. The more I tried to call time out, the more sessions we would have. The more my suicidality peaked, the more my therapist's anxiety peaked, thus necessitating more sessions or check-ins. Things weren't going well and we didn't know why. My therapist, I felt, was getting too attached to me and I wanted no part of it, yet I was developing feelings toward her, as well. But we didn't talk about it.

I don't know who came up with the idea of seeing a consultant to see how to progress. We needed an intervention before we both drove each other apart.

This was sometime in 2009. Trouble was, we were conflicted about what kind of consultant we needed. She thought a trauma specialist might help, but I wasn't sure. I read this specialist's website and papers, but she kind of scared me. I do not get along with the word "trauma". To me, it is the scariest word in the English language. And the last thing I wanted was for someone to tell me that I had to deal with it if I was going to move forward. So this person was out, at least for the time being.

I had read about CBASP, Cognitive Behavioral Analytical System of Psychotherapy, as a treatment for resistant depression. I thought it might work for me. The trouble was there weren't any CBASP trained therapists in my area. The closest one was in Rhode Island and there was no guarantee this person would see me. So we left that on the table, as well.

Midnight Demon

Because my suicidality was ongoing, we decided that seeing a suicide specialist might be fitting. I had met someone at the 2008 AAS annual conference that had done my consult when I first was hospitalized for my medically serious attempt. I felt he might be a good guy to consult. When I called him, he had to decline as he no longer did consultant work, but he referred me to another clinician that did. Are you seeing a pattern here?

I had read some stuff by the guy he referred me to. His name is Dr. G, but I didn't make the connection until after the fact. I thought this might work out. My therapist was still practicing in Cambridge and this guy was right down the street from her office. It would be ideal for us.

He wanted to interview my therapist first, which I was fine with. I was a little scared, as I am always afraid that mentioning suicide would force me into the hospital. That had been the case for so long, that I was always fearful on how someone new was going to handle it. After my therapist met with him, she said that he was very interested in meeting me and would only discuss what he said after I met with him. I figured the chances of him hospitalizing me were slim after that.

I don't remember much about that first interview other than I was nervous, but he seemed like a typical analyst, complete with couch. We talked about my suicide episodes and about my work with Bozo, plus the normal history information. It took almost three sessions before he told us what his recommendations were. He had figured out that it was obvious both my therapist and I had feelings for each other and that there was a curious thing between us. If we (Bozo and I) didn't have a professional boundary, we might be close friends. He also picked up that she liked to talk a lot during sessions. So having her shut up and listen was going to be a challenge. Five years later, it still is, although when I tell her to shut up, she does…for a little while, at least. He also recommended she get to know me more and wanted some sessions with me as a sort of conjunctive therapy. I think I had close to five sessions. It helped a little bit, but his style was totally different than Bozo's. He was very reserved in his manner. He got that my pain should be taken care of and that I should be using any means necessary to decrease it. He liked the idea of using the psychache scale in sessions with Bozo and encouraged more transference. The hard part was remembering all he had to say. I was usually in a sleep-deprived state when I was with him as most of our sessions were in the early morning. I don't do mornings for this exact reason. But it was the only time he could fit me in so I had to grin and bear it, like I do most things. He thought that I didn't use the pain medication adequately because I had some fear that I didn't deserve it, that I felt I needed to be punished for whatever reason. He wanted to find out what those reasons were, but we never did. I decided that seeing two therapists was more stressful to me than seeing one so I stopped seeing the consultant, but brought his ideas to my therapist.

    We talked about it for a little while. I guess I still feel that I deserve to be in pain because I am a cruel person, that I must have done something evil to deserve it. I haven't figured out what I did yet. Some days I don't care and will take my medication. Other days, I let the pain linger longer than I should before I take it. I always hope that, by ignoring it, it will go away. It never does.

    What I took from the consultant was that this man, whom I have only met a few times, cared about me and wanted me to succeed in life. He saw the good in me, though *I* still could not see it. I guess all those years of my father telling me I am a nothing and am stupid does something to you. This consultant was the first male figure in my life that really tried to help me. We were able to talk about suicidality professionally, and it meant so much to be able to be open about my suicidal thoughts and not have to cover them up. Over the years, I still consult him on matters relating to my care. When Bozo finally moved to her final destination in Framingham, I decided that I needed someone a little closer. I went to him and asked him for a referral. There was no way I could see him because he wanted to stay on as a consultant. But because my insurance sucked, there were few people that he could refer me to. I was deeply saddened by this. I felt like I couldn't move past Bozo and I was right. The stars had aligned and there was no way I could terminate Bozo even if I wanted to. Bozo was here to stay, whether I liked it or not.

The consultant saw that we both cared for one another and that was a good thing to have in a therapeutic relationship. One thing I have learned in all my years of going to therapy is that if you don't have a good connection, building an alliance is not going to happen. As with any relationship, there has to be some give and take.

There came a time in my relationship with Bozo that we had to agree to disagree. It took many sessions for this to happen, but it did. Mostly, I would be the one to disagree with what she said rather than vice versa.

Closing Remarks

I never really thought ahead before. I found that if I did, it overwhelmed me too much so I always stuck with today or the hour or, sometimes, the minute because I had to. But now with this book, I am finding myself looking forward to the future more. It is a weird sensation. I am not saying this makes me less depressed. It makes me a little less suicidal or my suicidal thoughts float more than linger.

I have been in a weird space. I had a good session with my therapist and, for some reason, it put me in a good mood. Now I am wondering if I am hypomanic because I am in a good mood and have been up since 5. Things with the hypomania can spiral out of control quickly so if I am not my usual pessimistic self, I tend to worry.

My writing friend said that I should write about this weird sensation, but I am finding it difficult because it is not like me to think about the future. Usually, my future is pitch black because I don't have one. I know everyone does but, for a long time, I just didn't. Thinking about the future brought worry and anxiety. I had to get through today first and that was always difficult enough so I stopped thinking about future things. I still think that I can get my degree and my doctorate and be the therapist that I want to be. But those things are on the back burner and I don't know if I will ever achieve those goals. I know that I don't want to be old and gray, though. I have Alzheimer's on both sides of my family so I know there is a good chance that I might get it. I already am having trouble with memory. I often write things and I forget that I write them. I don't know if it is the dark side or just another part of me that was in the moment when I had these ideas. I am sure when I look back on this post, I am going to be like WTF. I wrote this?? That is so unlike me! And it is and that is what is weird.

My friend also thought that I don't reward myself because of my suicidality. I have been suicidal for so long that I don't think I can look past a month at a time without fearing losing my

Midnight Demon

life. It's like I am a Klingon and wake up every morning asking if this is the day I am going to die. People don't understand this. I know my family would be watching me like a hawk if they had any clue just how suicidal I have been the past few months. And the past two days, I have felt like I have been in an alternate reality or something because I'm thinking of my future. But this book that I am writing and slaving over has given me a different perspective. I want to see it published. I want to see it successful. If I sell a hundred copies, I will be happy…at least for a little while. But I didn't go on disability to be a successful writer. The bad stuff is still under the surface. I appear to be merry, cheerful, happy to the outside world, but I am tormented and my heart bleeds. Nothing can stop the bleeding. I thought that working on this book would help the ache and, to some degree, it has, but it is still there. I might not be feeling it a hundred percent of the time, all the time, but it is still there. I can't deny it any more than I can deny my foot pain that also is my nemesis. I am my own worst enemy. But today I can say that I am more a friend.

　　Though suicide has been a large part of my life, I still am able to resist it. This has not been easy to do as the feelings can be quite intense. But what has helped me get through it is having a crisis response plan. It is a plan that has a few steps in it. First, you identify what you are feeling or what is upsetting you. Second, you come up with alternatives to those thoughts and feelings. Third, if that doesn't work, you try and do something for thirty minutes, such as listen to music, comb your hair, write in your journal if you have one or start one if you don't, play games, take a long shower or soothing bath, etc. Then, if that doesn't work, repeat those things. I know it might sound a little mundane, but maybe you can think about things differently when doing them again. Fourth, if nothing works or you find yourself planning to do something, you call someone for help. It could be a friend, a therapist, or a suicide hotline. If you cannot get a hold of your therapist and you feel you're in imminent danger, go to the emergency room or call 911.

I felt like this book would be incomplete if it didn't have this information in it because it is so essential to saving lives. If you are in therapy and are suicidal, please show this to your therapist and work on ways to get better.

In my life, there has been a lot of pain, but the biggest thing that got me through it was the hope that tomorrow might be a better day. If I didn't have that, I would have nothing and I think I would have ended my life a long time ago.

Though I still think about killing myself, it has become my security blanket. It always is in the back of my mind whenever I am in a rough spot. One thing that I have learned is that you can feel whatever you want. It is what you do with those feelings that count. If you act on them, that puts you in danger. The hardest part is hanging on to let those feelings pass.

Even though my life is not always filled with blue skies and sunny days, I find that I get along better with gray, cloudy days because that is a better reflection on how I feel. Being true to oneself is the hardest thing to do.

Midnight Demon

Midnight Demon

References:

Jobes, D. A. (2006). *Managing suicidal risk: A collaborative approach*. New York, NY: Guilford Press.

Michel, K., & Jobes, D. A. (2011). *Building a therapeutic alliance with the suicidal patient*. Washington, DC: American Psychological Association; US.

Maris, R. W., Berman, A. L., & Silverman, M. M. (2000). *Comprehensive textbook of suicidology*. New York, NY: Guilford Press.

Shneidman, E. S. (1993). *Suicide as psychache: A clinical approach to self-destructive behavior*. Lanham, MD: Jason Aronson.

Jamison, K. R. (1993). *Touched With Fire*. New York: Free Press Paperbacks.

Styron, W. (1990). *Darkness Visible*. New York: Vintage

www.ingramcontent.com/pod-product-compliance
Lightning Source LLC
Chambersburg PA
CBHW051707170526
45167CB00002B/565